STUDY GUIDE TO ACCOMPANY

COMPREHENSIVE MEDICAL ASSISTING

ADMINISTRATIVE AND CLINICAL COMPETENCIES

Sixth Edition

Virginia Busey Ferrari, MHA, BA, CEHRS (NHA)

Julie A. Morris RN, BSN, CBCS, CCMA (NHA), CMAA (NHA)

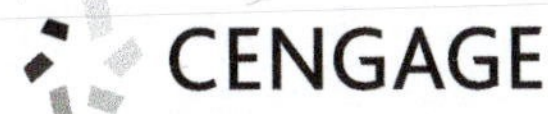

Australia • Brazil • Mexico • Singapore • United Kingdom • United States

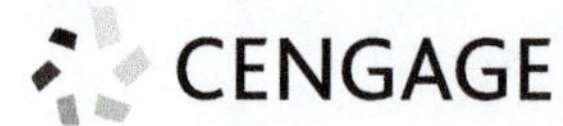

***Study Guide to Accompany Comprehensive Medical Assisting: Administrative and Clinical Competencies*, Sixth Edition**
Virginia Busey Ferrari, Julie A. Morris

SVP, GM Skills & Global Product Management: Jonathan Lau

Product Director: Matthew Seeley

Product Team Manager: Stephen Smith

Senior Director, Development: Marah Bellegarde

Product Development Manager: Juliet Steiner

Senior Content Developer: Lauren Whalen

Product Assistant: Mark Turner

Vice President, Marketing Services: Jennifer Ann Baker

Marketing Manager: Jessica Cipperly

Senior Production Director: Wendy Troeger

Production Director: Andrew Crouth

Senior Content Project Manager: Thomas Heffernan

Senior Art Director: Jack Pendleton

Media Producer: Jim Gilbert

Cover image(s): My Portfolio/Shutterstock.com
Vikpit/Shutterstock.com
Svetlana_Okeana/Shutterstock.com

For product information and technology assistance, contact us at
Cengage Customer & Sales Support, 1-800-354-9706
or support.cengage.com.

For permission to use material from this text or product, submit all requests online at **www.cengage.com/permissions.**

Library of Congress Control Number: 2017930060

ISBN: 978-1-305-96485-3

Cengage
200 Pier 4 Boulevard
Boston, MA 02210
USA

Cengage is a leading provider of customized learning solutions with employees residing in nearly 40 different countries and sales in more than 125 countries around the world. Find your local representative at: **www.cengage.com.**

To learn more about Cengage platforms and services, register or access your online learning solution, or purchase materials for your course, visit **www.cengage.com.**

Printed at CLDPC, USA, 05-21

CONTENTS

TO THE LEARNER

This Study Guide is part of a dynamic learning system that will help reinforce the essential competencies you need to enter the field of medical assisting and become a successful, multiskilled medical assistant. It has been completely revised to challenge you to apply the chapter knowledge from *Comprehensive Medical Assisting: Administrative and Clinical Competencies*, Sixth Edition, to develop basic competencies, use critical thinking skills, and integrate your knowledge effectively.

STUDY GUIDE ORGANIZATION

The Chapter Assignment Sheets are divided into the following sections: Vocabulary Builder, Learning Review, Certification Review, Learning Application, and Attributes of Professionalism. The content of the Study Guide has been designed to give you a creative and interpretive forum to apply the knowledge you have learned, not simply to repeat information to answer questions. Realistic simulations appear throughout the Study Guide that reference the characters in the textbook. This gives the material a real-world feel that comes as close as possible to your future experiences in an ambulatory setting. Clinical principles, such as infection control, communication, and patient education, are repeatedly reinforced through simulation exercises that require the ability to use your knowledge effectively and readily.

COMPREHENSIVE EXAMINATION

Feel certain that each procedure and concept you master is an important step toward preparing your skills and knowledge for the workplace. A final comprehensive examination is presented at the conclusion of the Study Guide, covering all the essential topic areas that medical assisting graduates must master. This examination has 200 questions and provides excellent practice for national certification examinations.

FINAL THOUGHTS

The textbook, Study Guide, and Competency Checklists have all been coordinated to meet the core objectives. Review the Learning Outcomes at the beginning of each chapter in the textbook before you begin to study; they are a road map that will take you to your goals.

Remember that you are the learner, so you can take credit for your success. The instructor is an important guide on this journey, and the text, Study Guide, and Competency Checklists are tools—but whether or not you use the tools wisely is ultimately up to you.

Evaluate yourself and your study habits. Take positive steps toward improving yourself, and avoid habits that could limit your success. Do family responsibilities and social opportunities interfere with your study? If so, sit down with your family and plan a schedule for study that they will support and to which you will adhere. Find a special place to study that is free from distraction.

Because regulations vary from state to state regarding which procedures can be performed by a medical assistant, it will be important to check specific regulations in your state. A medical assistant should never perform any procedure without being aware of legal responsibilities, correct procedure, and proper authorization.

As you pursue a wonderful career in medical assisting, make the most of your education and training.

Name ______________________ Date __________ Score __________

CHAPTER 1

The Medical Assisting Profession

VOCABULARY BUILDER

Misspelled Words

Find the words below that are misspelled; circle, them, and then correctly spell them in the space provided. Then insert the correct vocabulary terms from the list that best fit the statements below.

ambulatorie care setting	bachelor's degree	lisense
asociate's degree	competencie	practicum
attributes	compliance	professionalism

______________ ______________ ______________

______________ ______________ ______________

1. ______________ with standards and guidelines as stated by CAAHEP allows a medical assisting program to obtain programmatic certification.
2. Demonstrating ______________ is a key to being a successful medical assistant.
3. Medical assistants find employment most often in ______________.
4. Degrees available in medical assisting include ______________ and ______________ degrees.
5. Medical assistants are certified, but they do not hold a ______________.
6. Successfully obtaining certification demonstrates ______________ as a medical assistant.
7. An externship, or ______________, is an opportunity for the student to apply classroom knowledge and skills in a real-world medical setting.
8. Integrity, responsibility, and compassion are ______________ that are necessary for a medical assistant.

Matching

Match each term to its description.

________	1. Accreditation	A.	To make, invent, or arrange in an unplanned or spontaneous manner
________	2. Scope of practice	B.	Process whereby recognition is granted to an educational program for maintaining standards that qualify its graduates for professional practice
________	3. Improvise	C.	The ability to use one's hands skillfully
________	4. Proprietary	D.	Privately owned and managed facility, or a profit-making organization
________	5. Empathy	E.	Testimonials showing that a person is entitled to credit or has a right to exercise official power
________	6. Dexterity	F.	Ability to be objectively aware of and have insight into another's feelings or emotions
________	7. Credentialed	G.	The range of clinical procedures and activities that are allowed by law for a profession

LEARNING REVIEW

Short Answer

1. Define ethics.

____

2. What are the benefits of certification?

____

3. Describe continuing education activities.

____

____

4. List any five attributes of professionalism.

____

5. Describe the role of a Certified Medical Administrative Specialist.

____

____

6. Describe the history of the organization known as the American Association of Medical Assistants.

____

____

____

7. The U.S. Department of Labor, Bureau of Statistics, lists medical assisting as the fastest-growing allied health profession. Name eight settings where medical assistants are usually employed.

____

____

____

8. How does the American Association of Medical Assistants describe its members?

____

____

9. State the benefits of graduating from a program accredited by either CAAHEP or ABHES.

____

____

10. What are some of the benefits that medical clinics receive as a result of being a practicum site?

____

____

____

____

11. Write what each of the following abbreviations stands for.

AAMA: _______________

ACA: _______________

AMT: _______________

CCMA: _______________

CMAA: _______________

CMA: _______________

NHA: _______________

RMA: _______________

CERTIFICATION REVIEW

These questions are designed to mimic the certification examination. Select the best response.

1. Which term describes stepping into a patient's place, discovering what the patient is experiencing, and then recognizing and identifying with those feelings?
   a. Sympathy
   b. Association
   c. Flexibility
   d. Empathy

2. Which of the following statement(s) best describe(s) the professional medical assistant?
   a. The medical assistant has good written and oral communication skills.
   b. The medical assistant looks and acts professional at all times.
   c. The medical assistant is aware of the scope of practice and stays within the legal boundaries.
   d. The medical assistant assists the provider in all areas of the ambulatory care setting.
   e. All of the above

3. Which term describes a system of values that each individual has that determines perceptions of right and wrong?
   a. Laws
   b. Ethics
   c. Attributes
   d. Attitudes

4. In what way does a medical assistant display his or her professional attitude?
   a. By discussing his or her personal life at work because it is therapeutic for him or her
   b. By talking with his or her coworkers to help them with their problems
   c. By reminding his or her providers that he or she works only 7.5 hours per day
   d. By helping patients in a friendly and empathetic manner
   e. By doing a basic workload

5. Which of the following contributes to a professional appearance?
   a. Good nutrition and exercise
   b. Healthy looking skin, teeth, and nails
   c. Daily showering and use of deodorant
   d. All of the above

6. How does a medical assistant become involved with his or her professional organization?
   a. By attending local chapter or state meetings
   b. By attending a national conference or state convention
   c. By joining his or her national organization
   d. By offering to serve on a local, state, or national committee
   e. All of the above

7. Courses in a professional medical assisting program include a complement of general knowledge classes such as anatomy and physiology and which of the following?
   a. Assisting with minor surgery
   b. CPR
   c. Medical terminology
   d. All of the above

8. Which of the following terms describes regulation for health care providers that is legislated by each state and is mandatory in order to practice?
   a. Licensure
   b. Registration
   c. Certification
   d. Accreditation
   e. Both a and c

9. The period in which a student is able to apply his or her newly acquired skills as a medical assistant prior to graduation is known as which of the following?
   a. Practicum
   b. Residency
   c. Orientation
   d. None of the above

10. The medical assistant is educated in which of the following settings?
    a. Classroom
    b. Laboratory
    c. Surgical suite
    d. Radiology department
    e. Both a and b

LEARNING APPLICATION

Critical Thinking

1. Describe two benefits for medical assistants who join their professional organizations.

____

____

2. Explain what opportunities are available for medical assistants to improve their skills while on practicum (externship).

____

____

____

____

3. Many employers require credentialed medical assistants. Give two specific reasons why this is the case.

____

____

4. Explain two ways in which a certified or registered medical assistant can remain current with changes in health care and technology.

____

____

____

____

____

5. Research which of the credentials is most widely accepted in your geographic area. How would pursuing a different professional credential affect your ability to find employment?

____

6. Patients and providers prefer to have working for them professional medical assistants who have had the benefit of a formal education. Discuss the impact of this education on patients and employers. Why is it important to both groups?

Case Studies

CASE STUDY 1

During your course of studies to become a medical assistant, you have an opportunity to volunteer to help out at a multiprovider urgent care center downtown in a large city to gain some firsthand experience in a professional setting.

CASE STUDY REVIEW QUESTIONS

1. Would this opportunity be interesting to you? Would you want to volunteer in this professional setting?

2. Even though you are a volunteer, why is it important to look and behave like a professional?

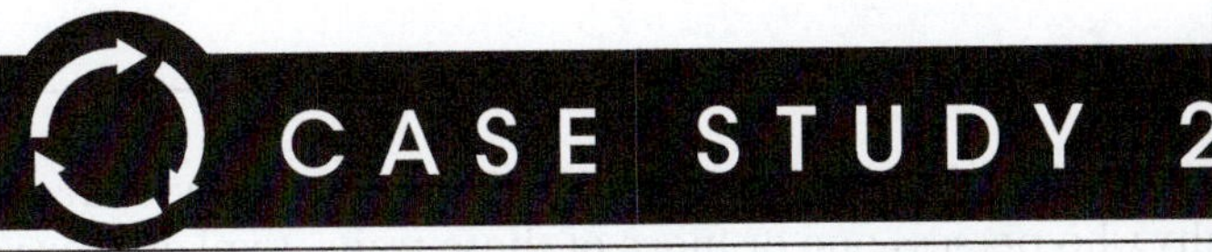

Linda Ludemann is preparing for her practicum. Linda is an excellent student, detail oriented, responsible, and professional in her dress and attitude. Linda is eager to experience her practicum with a large general practice or clinic with open hours built into the schedule for emergency patients, such as Inner City Health Care. Linda is intrigued by the idea of working with a group of providers and a diverse patient population where she can really work on improving her screening skills. Linda, however, is shy and quiet; she has difficulty meeting new people and relies on a core group of friends.

CASE STUDY REVIEW QUESTIONS

1. Is Linda really suited to practicum at Inner City Health Care? What are the potential advantages and disadvantages of this practicum placement?

2. What would be some ways in which Linda could overcome the difficulty she experiences when meeting new people?

3. Ease in working with diverse populations is just a small part of being a health care professional. What suggestions would you offer Linda in reaching her goal of professional growth?

4. Consider your own short- and long-range goals. How important is it to challenge yourself, personally and professionally, with experiences that contribute to your growth and knowledge? How can you use your practicum placement to work toward fulfilling your goals?

Role-Play

Assign the role of provider, clinic manager, and medical assistant to a group of students in your class. Role-play a roundtable discussion regarding the benefits of certification and the merits of each certification that is offered.

ATTRIBUTES OF PROFESSIONALISM

1. For each of the attributes listed in your textbook to describe a professional, identify individuals from your family, circle of friends, work, or community who possess one or more of those traits. Explain why you chose them.

2. Imagine your first day in your practicum. What will you wear? How will you prepare the night before? How will you look? Would you change your hairstyle? Makeup? Jewelry?

3. Review the listing of Attributes of Professionalism in Chapter 1. List the one attribute that you feel would be a challenge for you and write a short description regarding ways that you will begin to develop in that particular area. Now select the attribute that will be easiest for you to represent. List it and briefly explain why this attribute comes easily for you.

3. Discuss the importance of keeping personal and professional goals in perspective.

4. What would be Liz's best therapeutic response to Dr. Osborne?

ATTRIBUTES OF PROFESSIONALISM

Reflecting on the content you learned in this chapter, list some examples of the effects of stress/burnout on professionalism. How would you, in your position as a medical assistant, manage those effects in order to best interact with colleagues and patients? Cite examples.

2. Bill, who is 28 years old, comes for his annual checkup. When reviewing his social data sheet, you discover he is now living in an apartment and has a new phone number. He mumbles to you that his wife left him and won't let him see the kids. How will you respond therapeutically?

____

____

3. You try to be gentle and gracious with Edith. She is fragile and difficult to please. While positioning her for a radiograph, she sneers and says, "You are about the roughest person who ever cared for me." How will you respond therapeutically, and how will you control your body language?

____

____

____

____

4. When you report to Herb that his cholesterol is quite high and that the doctor wants to discuss medication and diet, he responds, "That is impossible; you must have made some mistake." Which defense mechanism is Herb using? How will you respond therapeutically?

____

____

Case Studies

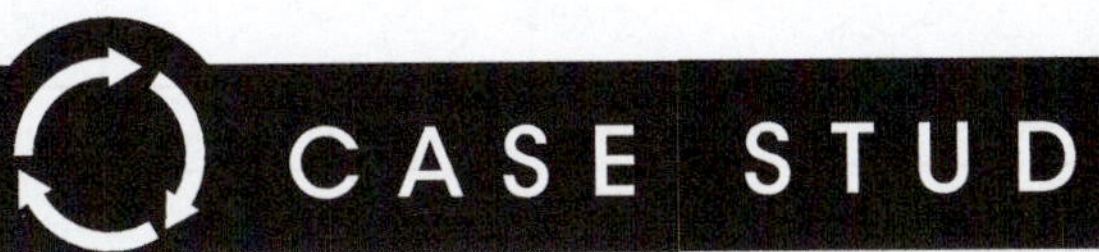

CASE STUDY 1

Wayne Elder arrives at Inner City Health Care for an examination to check on a recurrent ear infection that has been treated with antibiotics. Wayne, who has a slight intellectual disability and lives in a group home, is still reporting dizziness and pain in his right ear. He has come to the clinic by himself, taking a bus from his job as a part-time dishwasher. Wayne's boss asked him to return to the clinic because Wayne could not concentrate at work.

Nancy McFarland, RMA (AMT), who is a medical assistant at the clinic, discovers from Wayne that he has not been taking his medication properly; he stopped taking his pills once his ear began to feel better. She must politely ask Wayne to repeat himself several times before she can clearly understand his slurred speech, and she has difficulty holding his attention or maintaining eye contact.

Nancy conveys Wayne's situation to Dr. Ray Reynolds, who examines Wayne and gives him a new prescription for antibiotics, gently explaining the need to finish the entire prescription to get well. After Dr. Reynolds leaves the examination room, however, it is clear to Nancy that Wayne is still confused about why he must take the medication even after he begins to feel better. Nancy carefully explains to Wayne that the infection will continue to heal even though he no longer feels sick. To be sure he understands, Nancy asks Wayne to repeat to her what he must do and why; she then asks Dr. Reynolds to step in briefly to remind Wayne once more to complete the prescription.

CASE STUDY REVIEW QUESTIONS

1. How does the unequal relationship that exists between patients and health care professionals have an impact on the therapeutic communication between provider, medical assistant, and patient apply to the scenario in this case study?

2. How must medical assistant Nancy McFarland tailor her verbal and nonverbal messages to meet the abilities of her receivers: the provider and the patient?

3. How does Nancy use active listening? Which interview techniques are the most effective in facilitating therapeutic communication? Does nonverbal communication play a role?

4. Using Maslow's Hierarchy of Needs, discuss how the health care team meets Wayne's special needs resulting from his disability.

5. Do you think the medical assistant acted appropriately? What else could she have done? What should she not do in this situation?

Role-Play Exercises

Active listening is an important element of therapeutic communication. To practice active listening skills, role play as a patient and a medical assistant. Have the "patient" say each of the phrases below. The "medical assistant" should then rephrase each of the messages for verification from the sender and also include a therapeutic response. When you are finished role playing, write what you have said in response to each statement below.

1. "I don't know what to do. My father takes so many pills he can't remember which is the right one, so he ends up refusing to take any of them."

____

____

____

2. "I can't give you my insurance card because I lost it and I can't remember the name of the company, either. You've always taken care of this before."

____

____

3. "I can't help being worried. The doctor just suggested a referral for treatment at that hospital where somebody had their wrong foot operated on. What do you think?"

____

____

____

4. "I feel dizzy just thinking about having my blood taken. Do you really need to do it?"

____

____

ATTRIBUTES OF PROFESSIONALISM

Think about your own facial expressions and body language. Are you always portraying the message you want to send? List two situations in which you have been misinterpreted through your nonverbal communication, or situations in which you have misinterpreted someone else's message. Then think of a verbal message that could have helped make the situation more accurate. That is, explain what you could have said to the person to determine if he or she was really hearing the message you meant to send.

____

____

____

____

____

____

Name ______________________ Date ________ Score ________

CHAPTER 5

The Therapeutic Approach to the Patient with a Life-Threatening Illness

VOCABULARY BUILDER

Misspelled Words

Find the words below that are misspelled; circle them, and correctly spell them in the space provided. Then insert the correct vocabulary terms from the list that best fit the descriptions below.

durible power of attorney for health care	health care directive	palyative
______________	______________	______________

1. A ______________________ allows an individual to make decisions related to health care when the patient is no longer able to do so.

2. Before a patient becomes incapacitated, a ______________________ allows him or her to make decisions related to whether life-prolonging medical or surgical procedures are to be continued, withheld, or withdrawn, as well as if or when artificial feeding and fluids are to be used or withheld.

3. ______________________ care focuses on quality of life while relieving symptoms of pain and suffering alongside of or instead of disease-focused treatment.

LEARNING REVIEW

Short Answer

1. List five issues that are appropriate to discuss with a patient facing a life-threatening illness.

____

____

2. The federal government passed the ________________________ in 1990, giving all patients receiving care in institutions that receive payments from Medicare and Medicaid written information about their right to accept or refuse medical or surgical treatment.

3. Explain what each of the letters in the acronym *TEAR* means as it relates to the grieving process.

____

____

____

____

4. What is the best therapeutic response to a patient with a life-threatening disease?

____

____

____

____

____

____

____

____

CERTIFICATION REVIEW

These questions are designed to mimic the certification examination. Select the best response.

1. Your patient's culture influences which of the following?
   a. His or her views about illness
   b. His or her views about pain and treatment
   c. His or her views about death
   d. All of the above

2. Your patient has just been diagnosed with a life-threatening illness. She tells you that she would much rather die quickly than to suffer through this disease. She asks you not to say anything about her comment to the doctor. What is your best response?
   a. You have had quite a shock. I believe Dr. King would like to talk to you about those feelings. May I go get him for you?
   b. You, above anyone else, know what is best for your life.
   c. I know what you mean; I would feel the same way.
   d. Don't worry about that right now. Dr. King will give you medication to help with the pain.
   e. My grandfather had the same disease and it was very painful and difficult for him.

3. The health care directive and power of attorney for health care documents are legal in how many states?
   a. 10
   b. 25
   c. 5
   d. 50

4. The slowing of physical and mental responses, decreased alertness, withdrawal, apathy, and diminished interest in work are referred to as what?
   a. Passive-aggressive behavior
   b. Fight or flight
   c. Psychomotor retardation
   d. Mood swings
   e. Early onset dementia

5. Which of the following would be considered the strongest influence in managing the life-threatening illness of a patient?
   a. Health care team
   b. Family and those closest to the patient
   c. Social worker
   d. Hospice

6. The range of psychological suffering a patient may experience can lead to which of the following?
   a. Tachycardia
   b. Anorexia
   c. Agitation
   d. Insomnia
   e. All of the above

7. What do patients fear more than anything else when facing a life-threatening illness?
   a. Pain and loss of independence
   b. Dementia
   c. Financial issues
   d. Becoming addicted to some medications

8. When caring for individuals with life-threatening illnesses, which of the following would be helpful to remember?
   a. That family members have the strongest influence on patients
   b. That pain must be considered within a cultural perspective
   c. That choices and decisions regarding treatment belong to the patient
   d. To involve patients in the decision-making process
   e. All of the above

9. While no two individuals respond to a life-threatening illness in the same way, which of the following is the most common emotion?
   a. Displacement
   b. Denial
   c. Depression
   d. Assimilation

10. Referrals to community-based agencies or service groups may include which of the following?
    a. Health departments
    b. Social workers
    c. Hospice
    d. AIDS and cancer volunteers
    e. All of the above

LEARNING APPLICATION

Critical Thinking

1. Discuss with a friend what cultural influences might affect each of you if you were facing a life-threatening illness. What choices would each of you make?

2. Discuss with a classmate your concerns in dealing with patients with a life-threatening illness. Would you choose to work where you seldom lost a patient to a life-threatening illness? If so, what are your reasons?

3. A danger in having a fair amount of knowledge about life-threatening illnesses and the grief that accompanies them can be that we hope to be able to "fix" everything. With a friend, discuss the following statement made by Dr. Kübler-Ross: "Listen to the dying. They will tell you everything you need to know about when they are dying. And it is easy to miss." What does she mean? Why is it easy to miss?

4. What steps would you personally take to make certain you do not burn out from caring for patients with a life-threatening illness?

Case Studies

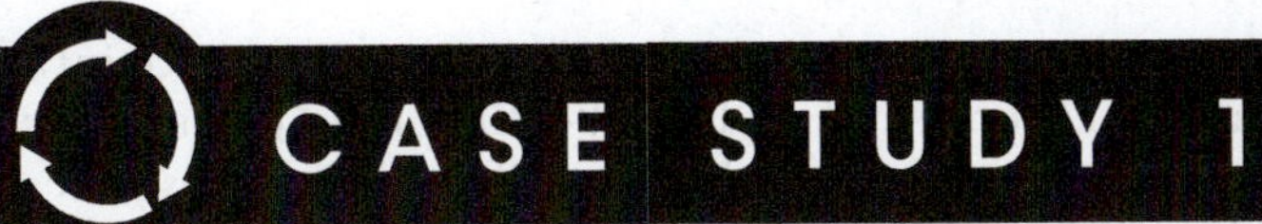

Jaime Carrera, a Hispanic man in his late 20s, is brought to Inner City Urgent Care by co-workers when he injures his head in an accident at a construction site where he is working. His head is bleeding profusely. As Jaime's co-workers watch the health care team implement Standard Precautions for infection control, one of them, his own shirt and hands covered with Jaime's blood, pulls the medical assistant aside and whispers frantically, "What are you doing? Does he have AIDS?"

CASE STUDY REVIEW QUESTIONS

1. What is the best therapeutic response of the medical assistant?

____

____

____

____

____

____

2. On what criteria do you base this response as the best therapeutic approach?

____

____

____

____

Role-Playing Exercises

With another student, role play the following scenarios as medical assistant and patient. What is the medical assistant's appropriate therapeutic response or action?

1. The patient's wife has just found out that her husband has end-stage renal disease. She tells the medical assistant that under no circumstances should her husband be informed about the prognosis.

____

____

____

2. The patient has been diagnosed with HIV. The medical assistant knows the patient is estranged from his or her family.

____

____

____

ATTRIBUTES OF PROFESSIONALISM

If you have had a family member that has faced a life-threatening issue, how has that experience influence your decision making? Reflect on how other medical professionals did or did not exhibit the Attributes of Professionalism when caring for your family member or friend. Describe how that experience influences your professionalism and attitude. What changes, if any, would you make in how you would treat patients experiencing similar circumstances?

Name ______________________ Date __________ Score __________

CHAPTER 6

Legal Considerations

VOCABULARY BUILDER

Misspelled Words

Find the words below that are misspelled; circle them, and correctly spell them in the spaces provided. Then insert the correct vocabulary terms from the list that best fit the descriptions below.

administer
administrative law
ajents
alternative dispute resolution
arbetrasion
civil law
common law
constitutional law
contract law
criminil law
deposition
despense
discovery
durable power of attorney for health care
emanciated minors
expert witness
expressed contract
feliny
implied consent
incompetence
lible
litigation
malfeasance
malpractice
mature miners
neglegance
noncompliant
plaintiff
risk management
slander
statutory law
subpena
tort

______________________ ______________________ ______________________
______________________ ______________________ ______________________
______________________ ______________________ ______________________
____

1. ______________________ Establishes agencies that are given power to enact regulations having the force of law

2. ______________________ Law that includes 27 amendments, 10 of which are the Bill of Rights

3. ______________________ Minors younger than 18 years who are free of parental care and are financially responsible, married, become parents, or join the armed forces

4. ______________________ Body of laws made by states; examples include medical practice acts, or laws, that regulate the practice of medicine, such as licensure and standards of care

5. ______________________ Describes failure to follow a required command or instruction

6. ______________________ A provider or health care professional who testifies in court; one who has enough knowledge and experience in a field to be able to testify to what is the reasonable and expected standard of care

7. ______________________ The failure to exercise the standard of care that a reasonable person would exercise in similar circumstances

8. ______________________ Person who brings charges in a civil case

9. ______________________ Medical assistants are considered this for their employers

10. ______________________ Occurs when there is a life-threatening emergency, or when the patient is unconscious or unable to respond; also occurs in more subtle ways such as when a patient tilts her head back and opens her eyes wide for instillation of medicated eye drops from a medical assistant without any verbal instructions to do so

11. ______________________ Professional negligence or the failure of a medical professional to perform the duty required of the position, causing injury to another

12. ______________________ Court order to appear, provide records, or both

13. ______________________ Person against whom charges are brought

14. ______________________ False and malicious spoken words. For example, a patient says loudly in the reception area of Inner City Health Care, filled to capacity with waiting patients, "Dr. Reynolds should retire—I know he's not up on the latest medical techniques."

15. ______________________ False and malicious writing about another, such as in published materials, pictures, and media. For example, a medical assistant documents in the patient's record, "Jim Marshall is a ruthless, rude man who is very full of himself. Be careful around him."

16. ______________________ A 17-year-old student who lives with his or her parents

17. ______________________ Actions that make the medical assistant and the employer less vulnerable to litigation

18. ______________________ Lawsuit

19. ______________________ Written or verbal contract that describes exactly what each party in the contract will do

LEARNING REVIEW

Identifying Civil and Criminal Law

Identify whether the following actions fall under the domain of civil law (CV) or criminal law (CM).

_______ A. A provider is siphoning narcotics from an urgent care center's locked drug cabinet and continuing to treat patients while under the influence of the drugs.

_______ B. A woman in the advanced stages of breast cancer sues her insurer when it refuses to provide benefits for a bone marrow transplant.

_______ C. A clinic manager steals, or embezzles, funds from the medical practice.

Short Answer

1. List and define the four Ds of negligence.

____

____

____

____

2. Before any invasive or surgical procedure is performed, patients are asked to sign consent forms, which become a permanent part of the medical record. What four things must the patient know to give informed consent?

____

____

____

____

3. The unauthorized touching of one person by another is called _______________________.

4. The federal government established laws in 1968 to allow people to make a gift of all or part of their body after death; it is known as the _______________________.

5. The law mandates that the proper authorities be informed of certain harms and injuries, such as *(circle all that apply)*:
   a. Rape
   b. Gunshot and knife wounds
   c. Child abuse
   d. Elder abuse
   e. Transmittable or contagious diseases

6. What term is used now in place of *domestic violence* and what does it mean? Why was this change made?

____

____

____

____

7. What is the difference between an advance directive and a POLST form?

____

____

____

____

8. In the case of Good Samaritan laws, does the medical assistant have any liability if an injury occurs after performing first aid?

____

____

____

CERTIFICATION REVIEW

These questions are designed to mimic the certification examination. Select the best response.

1. The Patient Self-Determination Act, which includes health care directives, ensures that patients are able to do what?
   a. Choose their own providers
   b. Control their own health care decisions
   c. Have guaranteed confidentiality
   d. Have health care benefits

2. Which of the following covers the relationship between providers and their patients?
   a. Informed consent
   b. Locum tenens
   c. Medical ethics
   d. Criminal law
   e. Civil action

3. What does *res ipsa loquitur* mean?
   a. The thing speaks for itself
   b. The provider is ultimately responsible
   c. The record must be opened in court
   d. Patients have a right to their records

4. Which of the following correctly identifies the four Ds of negligence?
   a. Duty, derelict, danger, damage
   b. Danger, duty, direct cause, disaster
   c. Duty, derelict, direct cause, damage
   d. Disaster, damage, direct cause, danger
   e. Direct cause, duty to inform, damage, despair

5. What is a 17-year-old individual who is in the navy considered to be?
   a. *Respondeat superior*
   b. An emancipated minor
   c. Privileged
   d. A naval dependent

6. What does *respondeat superior* (a Latin term) mean?
   a. Providers are responsible for their employees' actions
   b. The thing speaks for itself
   c. Obey your superior
   d. Breach of duty of care
   e. The master is not required to answer
7. What must the inventory of controlled substances include?
   a. List of the name, address, and DEA registration number of the provider
   b. Date and time of inventory
   c. Signature of the individual taking inventory
   d. All of the above
8. Under what circumstances is a provider legally bound to treat a patient?
   a. Until the patient breaks an appointment
   b. Until the patient does not have health insurance
   c. Until the patient cannot get a referral
   d. Until the patient no longer needs treatment
   e. Until the maximum insurance reimbursement has been reached
9. If suspicion of child abuse is aroused, what should the health care provider do?
   a. Send the patient home
   b. Treat the child's injuries
   c. Inform the parents of the child's diagnosis and that it will be reported to the police and social services agency
   d. Both b and c
10. When a patient is asked to walk across the hall to the treatment room while wearing only a patient gown and is in full view of other patients, what is this considered?
    a. A HIPAA violation
    b. Implied consent
    c. Invasion of privacy
    d. Defamation of character
    e. Express witness

LEARNING APPLICATION

Critical Thinking

1. Do you have a living will or advance directive? Why or why not? Identify to a family member or loved one what your wishes might be if you were seriously injured in an accident and were still in what appeared to be an irreversible coma after 10 months.

   ____

   ____

   ____

   ____

   ____

2. Discuss the medical assistant's obligations in regard to public duties.

3. Describe Good Samaritan laws. What must a medical assistant and any other health care professional remember when giving first aid at the scene of an accident?

4. Describe three types of abuse. Tell what your role as a medical assistant is when Juanita brings her 3-year-old son Henry to the clinic. Henry has bruises on his face and chest and appears quite frightened when you approach him. While you prepare Henry for the pediatrician's examination, Juanita's answers to your questions seem evasive.

4. Identify the types of providers or medical specialties most likely to administer and dispense as well as prescribe controlled substances.

Case Studies

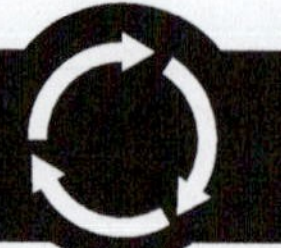

CASE STUDY 1

Dr. Mark King has just completed a routine physical examination of Abigail Johnson. Mark asks Nancy McFarland, RMA (AMT), to administer a flu shot to Abigail before the patient leaves the clinic. Abigail, an older African American woman, is accompanied by her daughter. When Nancy starts the process of administering the flu vaccine, Abigail says, "Is that a flu shot? They make me sick. I don't want it." Abigail's daughter says, "Yes, she does want it. Go ahead and give it to her." Abigail begins to laugh. "Okay," Nancy says, "may I give you the vaccination?" Abigail says nothing, but she rolls up her sleeve. As Nancy administers the parenteral injection, the older woman looks up at her seriously and says, "I didn't want any flu shot. My daughter makes me get it every year." However, Abigail does not withdraw physically.

CASE STUDY REVIEW QUESTIONS

1. What errors were made that could leave the medical assistant and provider vulnerable to litigation?

2. How might the errors leave the health care professionals open to potential lawsuits?

3. How could the errors have been avoided through effective risk management techniques?

CASE STUDY 2

Dr. Mark King is going over the daily list of scheduled patients with Ellen Armstrong, CMAS (AMT). They are standing at the front desk close to the reception area, and several patients are waiting for the first appointments of the day. Dr. King's eyes move down the list and stop over the name Mary O'Keefe. "Mary O'Keefe," he mutters, "she's so neurotic and pestering. It's a small wonder her husband hasn't left her yet; just wait till they have that third child … I don't think I have the patience for Mary today."

CASE STUDY REVIEW QUESTIONS

1. What errors were made that could leave the medical assistant and provider vulnerable to litigation?

2. How might the errors leave the health care professionals open to potential lawsuits?

3. How could the errors have been avoided through effective risk management techniques?

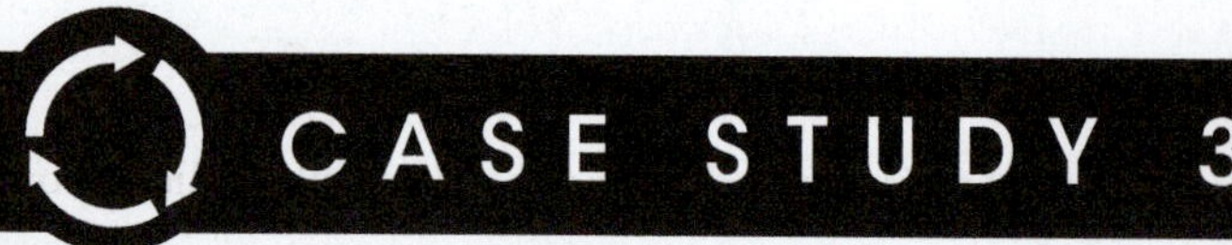

CASE STUDY 3

Lydia Renzi, who has impaired hearing, with some residual hearing, comes to Inner City Health Care and has waived her right to a certified sign language interpreter as provided under the Americans with Disabilities Act (ADA). She is at the clinic today with recurrent vaginal discharge. Lydia is diagnosed by Dr. Angie Osborne with candidiasis, a yeast infection caused by the fungus *Candida albicans.* Angie prescribes a vaginal suppository and asks Gwen Carr, CMA (AAMA), to give Lydia instructions for using the prescription. Lydia wears a hearing aid and has trouble understanding Gwen, who is soft spoken. Gwen is also standing against a brightly lit window, and Lydia has trouble seeing her face. Lydia writes on a pad she has brought with her, "Is this a sexually transmitted illness?" In frustration, Gwen begins shouting, "You just have a yeast infection; it's not like you have herpes or anything." At that moment, another medical assistant, Joe Guerrero, CMA (AAMA), is escorting a male patient past the open door of the examination room. Both men turn their heads away, though it is clear that they have overheard.

CASE STUDY REVIEW QUESTIONS

1. What errors were made that could leave the medical assistant and provider vulnerable to litigation?

____

____

2. How might the errors leave the health care professionals open to potential lawsuits?

____

____

3. How could the errors have been avoided through effective risk management techniques?

____

____

____

____

____

Role-Play Exercises

1. Apply the Patients' Bill of Rights related to treatment given the following circumstance. Pair up with a classmate, with one student playing the role of the medical assistant, and the other playing the role of the patient. The medical assistant must cite legal considerations in his or her response to the patient and display Attributes of Professionalism.

   SCENARIO: The primary care provider (PCP) instructs the medical assistant to contact a patient in regards to returned blood work indicating that additional chemotherapy is warranted. The medical assistant makes the call, but is informed by patient that there will be no more chemotherapy: "Enough is enough. I'm hoping for some quality of life for as long as I have left."

   ____

   ____

   ____

   ____

2. Report an illegal activity in the health care setting following proper protocol.

   SCENARIO: Log on to the Internet and review various news articles regarding the Veteran's Administration health care system scandal in 2014. Several "whistleblowers" came forward to disclose the illegal activity of using hidden wait lists. Use this (or a similar) scenario such as a colleague taking drug samples from the office for personal use, a colleague taking cash from the patient co-pay receipts, a provider or colleague injecting the wrong medication into a patient, a medical assistant or provider routinely billing for services not performed, a HIPAA violation, and so on. Pair up with a classmate and take turns role-playing reporting the illegal activity per proper protocol.

ATTRIBUTES OF PROFESSIONALISM

Have you ever been in a situation in which you were asked to disclose information about another person that might have been considered confidential? Or have you ever been told confidential information? If this has happened, what should you have done or said? If it happens in the future, what will you do or say?

____

____

____

____

____

____

Name ______________________ Date __________ Score __________

CHAPTER 7

Ethical Considerations

VOCABULARY BUILDER

Misspelled Words

Find the words below that are misspelled; circle them, and correctly spell them in the spaces provided. Then insert correct vocabulary terms from the list that best fit into the descriptions below.

bioethics	genetic enginering	macroallocation
criopreservation	in vetro fertlzation	microallocation
female genital mutilation	intimate partner violence	serrogate

_______________ _______________ _______________

_______________ _______________ _______________

1. _______________ Someone who substitutes for another
2. _______________ Biotechnology dealing with sophisticated medical research, diagnosis of disease, the production of medicines, or forensic documentation (DNA used in solving crimes)
3. _______________ Medical decisions related to scarce or limited resources made by Congress, health systems, agencies, and insurance companies
4. _______________ Medical decisions for scarce or limited resources made individually by providers and the health care team at the local level
5. _______________ Ethical issues dealing with all aspects of life and death
6. _______________ Occurs when an ovum is fertilized in a culture dish, allowed to grow, and then implanted into the uterus

LEARNING REVIEW

Code of Ethics Matching

The AAMA Code of Ethics presents five basic principles that medical assistants must pledge to honor as members of the medical assisting profession. For each situation presented, identify the AAMA ethical principle that applies.

A. Render service with full respect for the dignity of humanity

B. Respect confidential information obtained through employment unless legally authorized or required by responsible performance of duty to divulge such information

C. Uphold the honor and integrity of the profession and accept its disciplines

D. Seek to continually improve the knowledge and skills of medical assistants for the benefit of patients and professional colleagues

E. Participate in additional service activities aimed toward improving the health and well-being of the community

_____ 1. Marilyn Johnson, CMA (AAMA), in conversation with co–clinic manager Jane O'Hara, RMA (AMT), refuses to speculate about whether a diagnosis of AIDS will be confirmed for patient Maria Jover.

_____ 2. Administrative medical assistant Karen Ritter joins a study group to prepare for the CMA (AAMA) certification examination as a method of securing her certification credentials, which must be updated every 5 years.

_____ 3. Clinical medical assistant Anna Preciado, RMA (AMT), agrees to speak to a group of high school students who are interested in pursuing a career in the medical assisting profession.

_____ 4. Liz Corbin, CMA (AAMA), politely reminds older adult patient Edith Leonard that she is a certified medical assistant, not a nurse, and assures Edith that she is qualified to perform the instillation of medicated eye drops ordered by Dr. Angie Osborne.

_____ 5. When patient Dottie Tate makes an appointment at Inner City Health Care for follow-up treatment of chronic back pain and a recent history of frequent falls, Joe Guerrero, CMA (AAMA), arranges for a wheelchair to accommodate Dottie's office visit.

_____ 6. Karen Ritter volunteers at the local community office of Planned Parenthood on weekends.

_____ 7. Nancy McFarland, RMA (AMT), gently and kindly guides patient Wayne Elder, whose intellectual disability often causes him to become confused in unfamiliar settings, back to the proper examination room after she finds him wandering down the hallway in search of Dr. Ray Reynolds.

_____ 8. When filing a group of recent laboratory reports into the correct patient files, Ellen Armstrong, CMAS (AMT), takes care to complete the task quickly and efficiently. She performs the task at a private office station away from the general reception area and does not leave the charts open or unattended as she works.

_____ 9. Audrey Jones approaches clinic manager Shirley Brooks, CMA (AAMA), about opportunities for obtaining advanced training to become qualified to perform a wider array of clinical procedures in the ambulatory care setting.

_____ 10. Clinical medical assistant Wanda Slawson assists Dr. Mark Woo in the treatment of patient Rhoda Au, who has been diagnosed with lupus erythematosus. Wanda believes the patient is foolhardy when she rejects Dr. Woo's treatment plan of Western drug therapy in favor of an approach that includes traditional Chinese medicine. However, she respects the patient's heritage and right to choose her own health care.

Short Answer

1. Patient medical records are confidential legal documents. Name three instances, however, in which health professionals are allowed or required to reveal confidential patient information by law.

2. Issues of bioethics common to every medical clinic are *(circle all that apply):*
   a. Allocation of scarce or limited medical resources
   b. Genetic engineering or manipulation
   c. Abortion and fetal tissue research
   d. Many choices surrounding life, dying, and death

3. Individuals who are truly aware of their ethical power are able to *(circle all that apply):*
   a. Not compromise any procedure or technique
   b. Not ever put the patient at risk
   c. Hide the truth regarding a possible error

4. Allocation of scarce or limited medical resources may be related to *(circle all that apply):*
   a. Rationing of health care
   b. Denied services
   c. Advertising by health care professionals

5. In a case of suspected child abuse, the medical professional should *(circle all that apply):*
   a. Report the case
   b. Protect and care for the abused
   c. Treat the abuser, if known, as a victim also

6. List the five Ps of ethical power.

7. List the eight questions adapted from Stephen Covey's book that can be used as guidelines for making ethical decisions.

8. List six abuse factors that constitute intimate partner violence. (Hint: Refer to Table 7-1.)

____

____

____

____

____

____

____

____

____

____

CERTIFICATION REVIEW

These questions are designed to mimic the certification examination. Select the best response.

1. The AAMA Code of Ethics includes all but which one of the following?
   a. We should render service with respect for the dignity of humanity.
   b. We should be paid an equitable salary/wage.
   c. We should respect confidential information.
   d. We should accept the disciplines of the profession.

2. Providers may choose who to treat but may not refuse treatment based on certain criteria. Which of the following is *not* true?
   a. Providers may not refuse to treat patients based on race, color, religion, or national origin.
   b. It is unethical for a provider to refuse to treat a patient who is HIV positive.
   c. Providers must inform a patient's family of a patient's death and not delegate that responsibility to others.
   d. Providers who know they are HIV positive should tell their patients.
   e. Providers should report unethical behaviors committed by other providers.

3. To whom do medical records and information contained in them belong?
   a. Patient
   b. Patient and family
   c. Provider and patient
   d. Provider

4. Once a provider takes a case, under which of the following circumstances can the provider refuse treatment to a patient?
   a. The patient did not pay for her last visit.
   b. Official notice is given from the provider to withdraw from the case.
   c. The patient was a no-show.
   d. The patient did not keep the last appointment.
   e. The patient has a communicable disease.

5. If a provider suspects that an HIV-seropositive patient is infecting an unsuspecting individual, what should he do?
   a. Make every attempt to protect the individual at risk
   b. Report the case to the CDC
   c. Dismiss the patient from the practice
   d. Notify the department of health

6. What is the main objective of hospice?
   a. To provide pain relief on an "as-needed" basis to a patient with a terminal disease or condition
   b. To reduce costs for end-of-life care
   c. To make patients comfortable and as free from pain as possible and to allow them dignity in their deaths
   d. Provide patients with the directive of Do Not Resuscitate
   e. Allow families to make the end-of-life decisions that meet all family members' needs and resources

7. What should providers who know they are HIV positive do?
   a. Refrain from any activity that would risk transmission of the virus to others
   b. Wear a mask
   c. Inform the patients
   d. Retire

8. Revealing information about patients without consent may be done under what circumstance?
   a. When required by law, such as knife and gunshot wounds
   b. When sharing information anonymously across the Internet
   c. When reporting to a spouse the details of the patient's end-of-life decisions
   d. For the purpose of genetic manipulation and stem cell research
   e. All of the above

9. *Roe v. Wade* refers to guidelines for what?
   a. Artificial insemination
   b. Surrogacy
   c. Abortion
   d. Fetal tissue transplant

10. Decisions made by Congress, health systems agencies, and insurance companies regarding scarce or limited resources are termed what?
    a. Macroallocation
    b. Microallocation
    c. Bioethical dilemmas
    d. Exploitation
    e. Misallocation

LEARNING APPLICATION

Critical Thinking

1. A provider observes another provider put a patient at risk while under the influence of alcohol and does nothing about it. What would constitute ethical behavior?

2. A provider refuses to accept any more Medicaid patients for medical care. Is this the provider's right? Is it ethical? Why or why not?

3. A clinical medical assistant whispers to the administrative medical assistant, "There goes the guy with AIDS." How should the administrative medical assistant view this behavior?

4. A provider performs artificial insemination for a lesbian couple; however, the medical assistant refuses to participate or assist the provider. What are the ramifications of the medical assistant's behavior? Do you believe the medical assistant has a right to refuse?

Case Studies

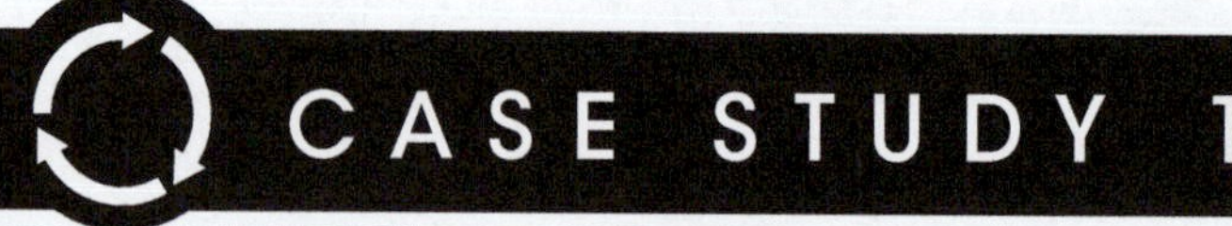

Lourdes Austen arrives at Inner City Health Care for her annual physical examination. It has been one year since Lourdes had surgery to remove a tumor in her breast by lumpectomy with axillary lymph node dissection, followed by a course of radiation. Lourdes's 1-year mammogram and follow-up examination with her surgeon and radiologist find no evidence of a recurrence of the cancer. Lourdes is a single woman in her late 30s. As Dr. King begins the routine physical examination, assisted by Nancy McFarland, RMA (AMT), Lourdes begins to cry. "I'm so happy to be alive," Lourdes says. "And so afraid of the cancer coming back. But I want to celebrate life. I've talked to my boyfriend about it and we want to get pregnant. What should I do?" Dr. King takes Lourdes's hand. "I know that living with cancer is hard. You are doing well. There are many things to consider...."

CASE STUDY REVIEW QUESTIONS

1. What bioethical dilemma exists in Lourdes's situation? In your opinion, is Lourdes's choice to become pregnant an ethical one?

2. How do deeply held beliefs and attitudes about parenthood and the role of women in our society have an impact on the patient's decision? How could these beliefs have an impact on the health care team's response to Lourdes?

3. What is Dr. King's best therapeutic response to Lourdes? What medical issues should the health care team consider if Lourdes becomes pregnant?

ATTRIBUTES OF PROFESSIONALISM

Identify how you are able to demonstrate the five Ps of ethical power in your own life. Do you think there is any overlap between the five Ps and the Attributes of Professionalism? Explain.

Name ______________________________ Date __________ Score __________

CHAPTER 8

Emergency Procedures and First Aid

VOCABULARY BUILDER

Misspelled Words

Find the key vocabulary words below that are misspelled; circle them, and correctly spell them in the spaces provided. Then insert the correct vocabulary terms into the sentences below. Not all vocabulary terms will be used.

anapylactic	crepitation	sprane
avultion	explicit	syncopy
cardiopulmonary resuscitation	hypothermea	treeage

______________________ ______________________ ______________________

______________________ ______________________ ______________________

1. After administering the antibiotic, the patient exhibited symptoms of ______________________ shock.
2. When a bone is fractured, there is often ______________________ at the site.
3. A ______________________ is an injury to a joint.
4. When the body temperature drops to a dangerous level, it is called ______________________.
5. Fainting is also known as ______________________.
6. ______________________ is abbreviated as CPR.
7. A system of determining which patients need care first based on the severity of their illness or injury is called ______________________.
8. The type of wound that results in the tearing away of the skin, subcutaneous fat and muscle from the bone is referred to as an ______________________.
9. ______________________ instructions are given to the patient for care of the wound after office surgery.

Matching I

Identify each of the following terms as an emergency condition (EC), an emergency or first aid procedure performed by health care professionals (EP), emergency equipment (EQ), or an emergency service provided to assist in emergency situations (ES).

_____ A. First aid

_____ B. Screening

_____ C. Syncope

_____ D. Shock

_____ E. Wounds

_____ F. Crash cart

_____ G. Occlusion

_____ H. Universal emergency medical identification symbol and card

_____ I. Hypothermia

_____ J. Chest compressions

_____ K. CPR

_____ L. Sprain

_____ M. Emergency medical service (EMS)

_____ N. Fracture

_____ O. Splints

_____ P. Strain

_____ Q. Rescue breathing

Matching II

Match each of the terms in Matching I with its definition below.

_____ 1. A break in a bone; there are several types, but all are classified as open or closed

_____ 2. A tray or portable cart that contains medications and supplies needed for emergency and first aid procedures

_____ 3. An injury to the soft tissue between joints that involves the tearing of muscles or tendons and occurs often in the neck, back, or thigh muscles

_____ 4. A break in the skin or underlying tissues, categorized as open or closed

_____ 5. Closure of a passage

_____ 6. An injury to a joint, often an ankle, knee, or wrist, that involves a tearing of the ligaments; most are minor and heal quickly; others are more severe, include swelling, and may not heal properly if the patient continues to put stress on the affected joint

_____ 7. A local network of police, fire, and medical personnel trained to respond to emergency situations; in most communities, the system is activated by calling 911

_____ 8. Identification sometimes carried by individuals to alert to any health problems they might have

_____ 9. Any device used to immobilize a body part; often used by EMS personnel

_____ 10. An extremely dangerous cold-related condition that can result in death if the individual does not receive care and if the progression of the condition is not reversed; symptoms include shivering, cold skin, and confusion

_____ 11. Fainting

_____ 12. The immediate care provided to persons who are suddenly ill or injured, typically followed by more comprehensive care and treatment

_____ 13. A condition in which the circulatory system is not providing enough blood to all parts of the body, causing the body's organs to fail to function properly

_____ 14. The combination of rescue breathing and chest compressions performed by a trained individual on a patient experiencing cardiac arrest

_____ 15. To assess patients' conditions and prioritize the need for care

_____ 16. Performed on individuals in respiratory arrest, this is a mouth-to-mouth (using appropriate protective equipment) or mouth-to-nose procedure that provides oxygen to the patient until emergency personnel arrive

_____ 17. The act of applying pressure to someone's chest in order to help blood flow through the heart in an emergency situation

LEARNING REVIEW

Short Answer

1. While awaiting the arrival of EMS, what aspects of the patient's condition should the medical assistant continuously monitor?

____

____

2. What five infection control measures can health care professionals follow to greatly reduce the risk for transmitting infectious disease when providing emergency care?

____

____

____

3. For each of the patient symptoms or conditions below, identify the type of shock that is most likely.

Patient Symptom/Condition	**Type of Shock**
Patient suffers heart attack	________________
Patient experiences severe infection after colon surgery	________________
Patient experiences reaction to food allergy	________________
Patient sustains an injury to the trachea	________________
Patient has serious head trauma	________________
Accident victim experiences extreme loss of blood	________________

4. A common procedure for treating closed wounds is to RICE them. What do the letters of this acronym stand for?

____

5. Match each type of open wound (incision, puncture, laceration, avulsion, abrasion) to its defining characteristics.

Characteristics	**Type of Open Wound**
A wound that pierces and penetrates the skin. This wound may appear insignificant, but actually can go quite deep	________
These wounds commonly occur to exposed body parts such as the fingers, toes, and nose. Tissue is torn off and wounds may bleed profusely	________
A wound that results from a sharp object such as a scalpel blade	________
A painful wound. The epidermal layer of the skin is scraped away	________
A wound that results in a jagged tear of body tissues and may contain debris	________

6. For each type of open wound, describe proper emergency concerns, care, and treatment.

____

7. Name three sources, other than heat, that can cause burns. For each, describe the proper emergency concerns, care, and treatment.

____

8. Musculoskeletal injuries, or injuries to muscles, bones, and joints, can be difficult to assess, especially for closed fractures. List five assessment techniques that health care professionals can use to determine the seriousness of musculoskeletal injuries.

____

9. Review the symptoms listed below, and in the space provided to the left of each symptom, indicate *MI* for symptoms of myocardial infarction and *CVA* for symptoms of stroke.

_______________ 1. Numbness on one side of the body

_______________ 2. Pain radiating down one or both arms

_______________ 3. Excessive perspiration

_______________ 4. Shortness of breath

_______________ 5. Mental confusion

_______________ 6. Loss of vision

_______________ 7. Jaw pain

_______________ 8. Severe headache

_______________ 9. Slurred speech

_______________ 10. Rapid, weak pulse

10. Identify the method of entry into the body for each of the following poisons.

_______________ 1. Carbon monoxide

_______________ 2. Insect stingers

_______________ 3. Chemical pesticides used in the garden

_______________ 4. Drain cleaner

_______________ 5. Poison oak

_______________ 6. Cleaning fluid fumes

CERTIFICATION REVIEW

These questions are designed to mimic the certification examination. Select the best response.

1. Which of the following is not an appropriate treatment for hypothermia?
   a. Give the victim warm liquids to drink
   b. Remove any wet clothing
   c. Rub the victim's skin vigorously to increase circulation
   d. Use warm water to warm the person if possible

2. Which of the following symptoms may be reported when a patient is in anaphylactic shock?
   a. Feeling a constriction in the throat and chest
   b. Having difficulty breathing
   c. Having swelling and tingling of the lips and tongue
   d. Feeling faint or dizzy
   e. All of the above

3. What is the appropriate method for application of a closed compress?
   a. Apply until the victim feels tingling
   b. Apply for 10 minutes, then off for 40 minutes
   c. Apply for 20 minutes, then off for 20 minutes
   d. Apply for at least 1 hour, then off for 2 hours

4. To control nosebleeds, the patient should be seated, the patient's head elevated, and the nostrils pinched for what period of time?
   a. 10 minutes
   b. 20 minutes
   c. 30 minutes
   d. 40 minutes
   e. 45 minutes

5. Your best response to a patient call regarding a poisoning or suspicion of poisoning is to advise the patient to do which of the following?
   a. Call the poison control center
   b. Take charcoal
   c. Drink milk
   d. Flush the mouth with water

6. Which of the following is the best treatment for patients who are experiencing a seizure?
   a. Restrain them
   b. Stick a tongue depressor in their mouth
   c. Protect from injury and care for them with understanding
   d. Stop the seizure
   e. Wrap them tightly in a blanket to retain body heat.

7. Which type of shock occurs as a result of overwhelming emotional factors such as fear, anger, or grief?
   a. Neurogenic
   b. Psychogenic
   c. Anaphylactic
   d. Septic

8. The type of burn that may result in an entrance and exit burn wound area is which of the following?
   a. Chemical
   b. Electrical
   c. Solar radiation
   d. Explosion
   e. Scalding liquids

9. Which of the following burn depth classifications is another name for third-degree burns?
   a. Superficial
   b. Full thickness
   c. Partial thickness
   d. Sunburns

10. The type of fracture often caused by falling on an outstretched hand that involves the distal end of the radius is referred to as which of the following?
    a. Greenstick
    b. Spiral
    c. Colles
    d. Implicated
    e. Compound

LEARNING APPLICATION

Critical Thinking

1. A teenaged patient, Myles Parris, has been recently diagnosed with epilepsy. When he arrived at the clinic for today's appointment, he stated that he felt "odd." He then began to seize. The front desk staff notified the medical assistant who was responsible for triage in the clinic and she responded immediately.
   a. What actions should the medical assistant take initially?

   ____

   ____

   b. List several underlying diseases besides epilepsy that can cause seizures.

   ____

2. Ms. Cosper, a 52-year-old woman, came into the clinic for a routine follow-up appointment for her diabetes. She suddenly lost consciousness and slumped over in her chair in the waiting room. What immediate steps should be taken by the medical assistant?

   ____

3. Describe the purpose of a crash cart and list five medications and five supplies that should be found there.

   ____

   ____

   ____

   ____

   ____

   ____

   ____

   ____

4. Recall three types of bandages and give examples of their use.

   ____

   ____

   ____

   ____

5. Describe the difference between first-, second-, and third-degree burns.

   ____

   ____

   ____

6. Recall and describe the four routes of entry for poisons.

7. Explain when, why, and the technique for utilizing abdominal thrusts and back blows in an emergency situation.

8. Your practice has just received Poison Help Stickers from the Department of Health and Human Services to distribute to the parents of your pediatric patients. Create an educational flyer regarding poison prevention.

Case Studies

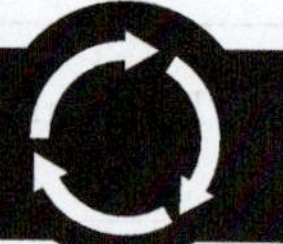

CASE STUDY 1

Mary O'Keefe calls Inner City Health Care in a panic. Gwen Carr, CMA (AAMA), answers the telephone.

Mary:	Oh my God, help me. I need Dr. King.
Gwen:	This is Gwen Carr. May I ask who's calling? What is the situation?
Mary:	It's my baby, oh God, get Dr. King.
Gwen:	Dr. King is unavailable, but we can help you. Now, tell me your name.
Mary:	It's Mary O'Keefe. Help me, I think my baby is dead.
Gwen:	Are you at home?
Mary:	Yes.
Gwen:	OK. Try to calm down. Speak slowly and tell me what's happened.
Mary:	My son Chris pried the plug off an outlet and he's electrocuted himself! [Mary cries.] He's just lying there. I'm so scared, if I touch him, will I electrocute myself? Oh my God, my baby, my baby. What should I do?

Gwen, who has been writing down the details on a piece of paper, motions to Thomas Myers, CCMA (NHA), and hands him her notes. Thomas immediately accesses the O'Keefe address from the patient database and uses another telephone to call EMS with the nature of the emergency situation and the address of the O'Keefe residence. Meanwhile, Gwen remains on the line with Mary. Dr. King is on rounds at the hospital this morning and will not be in the office for at least another hour. Gwen tells Mary, "Mary, we are calling EMS, and they will be there as soon as possible. In the meantime, I'm going to need you to focus and answer my questions, okay?"

CASE STUDY REVIEW QUESTIONS

1. What steps did the medical assistant take to screen the emergency situation?

2. What questions should Gwen ask Mary regarding the emergency situation?

3. What should the medical assistant do after EMS arrives and takes over emergency care? What follow-up procedures are necessary?

CASE STUDY 2

Lenore McDonell, a wheelchair-bound woman in her early 30s, experiences a serious laceration to the right arm sustained from a fall while performing an independent transfer from the examination table to her wheelchair. Joe Guerrero, CMA (AAMA), assists Dr. Winston Lewis in administering emergency care.

CASE STUDY REVIEW QUESTIONS

1. What Standard Precautions must the health care professionals follow before administering emergency treatment?

2. Joe and Dr. Lewis attempt to control Lenore's bleeding by applying a dressing and pressing firmly. When the bleeding does not stop, what two actions should the health care professionals perform?

3. The bleeding stops, and Joe applies a pressure bandage over the dressing. The patient is prone to fractures, and a radiograph will need to be taken. What is the next emergency procedure Dr. Lewis will perform? Why is this procedure necessary, and what equipment will the provider and medical assistant require?

4. Before applying a sling, what do the health care professionals check to be sure that the medical equipment used has not been too tightly applied?

5. What Standard Precautions will the health care team follow after the emergency treatment of the patient is successfully completed?

6. What information will the health care team include in documenting the procedure for the patient's medical record?

Screening Activity

In an urgent care setting, two or more patients may present at the same time with emergency symptoms. The order in which emergency patients will receive care depends on the health care professionals' abilities to screen patients' symptoms to determine who needs care most urgently. The following five patients present simultaneously on New Year's Eve at Inner City Urgent Care. Clinic manager Lynn Garrett, CMA (AAMA), is working the evening shift with Dr. Mark Woo. In what order will Lynn and Dr. Woo prioritize treatment? Number the patients 1 (most urgent) through 5 to correspond to the urgency of their conditions.

Patient	Urgency
Patient A presents with a gunshot wound to the leg that is bleeding severely. The patient is conscious but his pupils are dilated and he is unable to answer simple questions put to him by Lynn and Dr. Woo. He cradles his right arm and will not let anyone touch it, although there is no immediate evidence of an open wound to the arm.	___
Patient B, an elderly man, is brought in by his grandson. He describes debilitating chest pains, difficulty breathing, and nausea after eating a large family dinner. The patient's medical record indicates that he has a hiatal hernia, intervertebral disc disease, high blood pressure, and mild angina. The man is walking and speaking with moderate distress and is extremely anxious.	___

Patient C, a young woman, presents with her boyfriend. She appears to have multiple abrasions on her right palm and knee, with damage to the right knee and ankle joints sustained after a fall while on in-line skates. Both joints are swollen and painful.	____
Patient D, a man in his mid-30s, presents with the cotton tip of a swab stuck in his ear canal. Although the man feels a dull consistent pain in the ear, he says he has no trouble hearing. The outside of the ear appears normal, there is no bleeding evident, and the man appears annoyed but not distressed.	____
Patient E, a young woman, presents with a group of friends, all college students, with an eye injury sustained from a champagne cork. The cork, which had a metal covering over its tip, hit the patient's eye. The young woman's eye is red and tearing and she is experiencing severe pain in the eye.	____

ATTRIBUTES OF PROFESSIONALISM

1. On a scale of 1 to 5, rate your personal comfort in regard to the following emergency situations that medical assistants may find themselves involved with in an ambulatory or urgent care setting.

   1 = extremely uncomfortable

   2 = uncomfortable

   3 = somewhat comfortable

   4 = comfortable

   5 = very comfortable

   ___ Assisting in treatment of patients with injuries clearly sustained by an act of violence or abuse

   ___ Administering back blows and thrusts to a conscious infant

   ___ Performing rescue breathing on someone who has poor personal hygiene

   ___ Bandaging the open wound of a person with HIV infection

   ___ Caring for a person experiencing a seizure

   ___ Administering care to a patient who faints after venipuncture

   ___ Administering care to a patient in extreme pain

   ___ Administering care to a patient who is verbally abusive or uncooperative

2. On a scale of 1 to 5, rate your level of agreement with the statements that follow.

   1 = never

   2 = occasionally

   3 = sometimes

   4 = most of the time

   5 = all of the time

___ Life-threatening emergencies frighten me.

___ I respond well under pressure.

___ I am bothered by the sight of blood.

___ I lose my temper easily, becoming openly frustrated and angry.

___ I become frustrated and overwhelmed by feelings of helplessness in emergency situations.

___ I remain calm and clear-headed in emergency situations.

___ I forget about myself completely and focus on the emergency victim.

___ I am concerned about administering care in emergency situations in which danger to myself may exist when giving such care.

___ I am comfortable speaking to the family or friends of emergency victims.

3. Place an *X* beside the emergency interventions that fall into the scope of practice for a medical assistant.

___ Apply pressure to a bleeding wound

___ Start an IV in case the provider orders IV medication

___ Administer Benadryl orally per provider's order

___ Place the patient in Trendelenburg position

___ Suture a small laceration

___ Administer oxygen prior to the provider's assessment for a patient that is short of breath

___ Initiate CPR for a patient that has lost consciousness and is without a pulse

Name ______________________ Date ________ Score ________

CHAPTER **10**

Computers in the Medical Clinic

VOCABULARY BUILDER

Misspelled Words

Find the words below that are misspelled; circle them, and correctly spell them in the spaces provided. Then insert the correct vocabulary terms from the list that best fit the descriptions below.

electronic medical record	phisching	patches
cloud computing	hardware	practice management
erganomics	Internet	server

________________ ________________ ________________

________________ ________________ ________________

1. ________________ Scientific study of work and space, including factors that influence worker productivity and that affect workers' health
2. ________________ The physical equipment used by the computer system to process data, including input/output devices and CPU
3. ________________ The practice of attempting to acquire sensitive information (such as passwords or bank account numbers) by masquerading as a trusted source through email communication
4. ________________ Electronic patient records from a single medical provider, clinic, or hospital
5. ________________ A global computer network providing information and communication using interconnected networks
6. ________________ A category of software that deals with the day-to-day operations of a medical clinic

7. ______________________ Pseudo-computers connected to massive hard drives; in many networked systems they become the storage devices for the user workstations

8. ______________________ Storing program software on servers at a hosting company so that software download is available on demand

9. ______________________ Latest security fixes

LEARNING REVIEW

Short Answer

1. List the tasks that should be performed by members of the health care team when maintaining the computer.

____

____

2. What precautions must be taken to ensure that data are not lost during a power outage?

____

____

____

3. What are the three most common networks encountered in the medical clinic?

____

4. Name several hardware connections to a network.

____

5. Name several wireless connections to a network.

____

6. Name the two different techniques used by antivirus software to scan files to identify and eliminate computer viruses and malware.

____

____

7. List at least six of the defenses that should be used in protecting the health care facility's computer system.

____

____

____

____

____

____

8. What are the four fundamental elements of all computer systems?

____

9. What are the identifying characteristics of a secure site *(circle all that apply)*?
   a. Small padlock icon in the web browser window
   b. Site address: https://
   c. An *S* in the upper left corner of the screen
   d. Site address: http://

10. What is meant by "electronic medical record" and "electronic health record"? Distinguish between the terms.

____

____

CERTIFICATION REVIEW

These questions are designed to mimic the certification examination. Select the best response.

1. What is the drive that utilizes flash technology and is connected to the computer using a universal serial bus (USB 1.0, 2.0, or 3.0) port or higher performance USB serial port?
   a. USB thumb
   b. Cloud storage
   c. DVD drive
   d. Server

2. What step(s) should be followed when selecting software?
   a. Choose a knowledgeable vendor
   b. Develop a plan to determine what tasks will be computerized
   c. Seek input from staff and other medical clinics
   d. Select software available for each task should be identified and evaluated on a trial basis
   e. All of the above

3. The keyboard, mouse, digital camera, touch screen, scanners, laboratory test equipment, server files, CDs, and magnetic tape are examples of what element of a computer system?
   a. Central processing unit
   b. System software
   c. Output device
   d. Input device

4. What is the purpose of defragmenting?
   a. Removes fragments of information that you do not need anymore
   b. Removes old information no longer needed
   c. Removes blank spaces on the hard drive
   d. Removes software that you do not use
   e. Clears the cache stored in the computer

5. The category of computer that has very rapid processing speed through use of multiple processors connected in parallel and can fill a building is known as what?
   a. Mainframe
   b. Supercomputer
   c. Minicomputer
   d. Personal digital assistant
6. Which of the following are examples of output devices?
   a. Printers, fax machines, monitors
   b. Keyboards, mouses
   c. Scanners, electronic tablets
   d. Touch screens, digital cameras
   e. Cloud-based servers
7. What step(s) should be taken in the changeover to a computer system?
   a. Schedule during a down period, such as a long holiday or vacation period
   b. Introduce the new system while continuing to use the old system
   c. Transfer files and data; then when the staff are comfortable with the system and their computer skills, make the changeover
   d. All of the above
8. Manuals and licenses that define how many computers can use the software and how the program operates are known as what?
   a. Operating system
   b. System software
   c. Computer system documentation
   d. Application software
   e. All of the above
9. What type of drives are compact disks and digital video/versatile disks?
   a. Hard drives
   b. Optical drives
   c. Flash drives
   d. Tape drives
10. What is data storage device capacity often referred to as?
   a. Hardware
   b. Operating system
   c. Memory
   d. Algorithms
   e. Cloud-based

LEARNING APPLICATION

Critical Thinking

1. Assume you work in an ambulatory care setting that operates on a manual (paper) system. Identify what functions could be completed using a computer with an electronic health record program in the clinic.

2. The same clinic is now going to make the transition to a computerized system. What steps would you take to make the transition as smooth as possible?

3. Discuss the study of ergonomics and identify the steps to take in order to decrease or prevent computer-related injury.

4. Protecting a computer system from unauthorized access requires an in-depth defense. Using the Internet, identify as many defenses as you can find to protect the clinic. Prioritize the order of importance.

5. Your provider-employer has asked you to use the computer to research a particular medical topic. How do you proceed?

6. The provider-employer has informed the clinic manager that she has observed employees visiting Web sites not connected with clinic requirements and is concerned about the practice becoming widespread. You have been asked to prepare a draft guideline for a policy on business and personal Internet use on clinic equipment during business hours. You have been further told that the policy should not be totally prohibitive, but it does need to address performing personal tasks during business hours and exercising propriety in the sites visited.

Case Studies

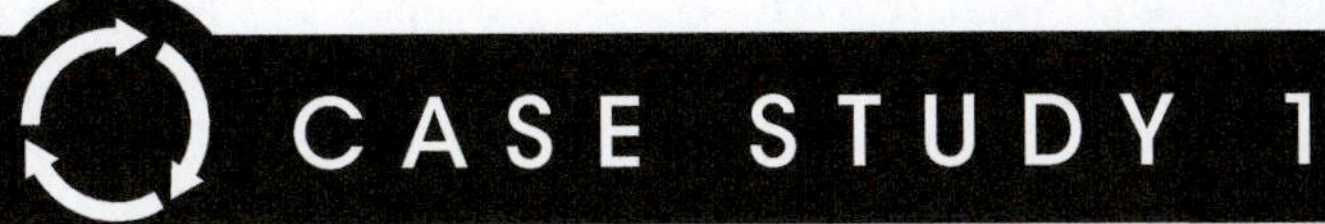

Due to an influx of patient volume, Inner City Health Care will have to hire more administrative staff and expand their office space. Three more computers have been installed, with updated software programs. Marilyn Johnson, CMA (AAMA), clinic manager, is trying to avoid any future safety issues in the workplace.

CASE STUDY REVIEW QUESTION

What factors should she take into consideration when setting up each workstation to be "ergonomically correct"?

____

____

____

____

____

____

____

____

____

ATTRIBUTES OF PROFESSIONALISM

Because we interact with and rely on computers (including smart phones) in almost all aspects of our personal lives and in the work environment, think about the Attributes of Professionalism and how they affect your personal and professional communications. Are you active on social networks? Which one(s) and how often? Look at your recent posts and posts of others and determine if they would be considered professional. What actions, if any, would you take regarding your social media account(s)? Does your use of a smart phone in the medical clinic violate HIPAA? Why or why not?

____

____

____

____

____

____

Name ______________________ Date __________ Score __________

CHAPTER 11

Telecommunications

VOCABULARY BUILDER

Misspelled Words

Find the words below that are misspelled; circle them, and correctly spell them in the spaces provided. Then fill in the blanks in the following paragraph with the appropriate terms. (Hint: Not all terms will be used.)

answering services	encryption	Good Samaritan laws
articulate	enunciation	jargine
automated routing unit	etiquette	modulated
buffer words	faximile	screening

______________________ ______________________ ______________________

______________________ ______________________ ______________________

When speaking on the telephone, medical assistants must use proper telephone __________, which means being courteous and professional to others. To ensure that listeners understand what is said, proper __________, or saying the words clearly, is important. Simple terms rather than medical __________ promote mutual understanding rather than confusion. The use of slang words and expressions is considered unprofessional and disrespectful. Proper pronunciation of all words in a carefully __________ voice will also help people understand what you are saying, especially non–English-speaking people. Good communication skills are of real benefit to a medical assistant when using the telephone and when speaking directly to patients.

Matching

Match the following devices or services with the corresponding descriptions.

______ 1. Answering service

______ 2. Cellular phone

______ 3. Automated routing unit

A. Takes calls when the clinic is closed

B. Sends a message via computer networks to an electronic mailbox located in another person's computer

C. A portable telephone

______ 4. Fax D. A document sent over telephone lines from one facsimile machine or modem to another

______ 5. Email E. A system that allows callers to reach specific people or departments by pressing a specified number on a touch-tone telephone

LEARNING REVIEW

Short Answer

1. Many hospitals and ambulatory care settings have telephone systems to manage heavy telephone traffic; these are called ____________________.
2. No call should be left unattended for more than ______ seconds.
3. What is the difference between enunciation and pronunciation?

____

4. Name the three different types of Voice-over-Internet Protocol (VoIP) services in use.

____

5. List three advantages of email and three disadvantages of email.

Advantages:

____

____

____

____

Disadvantages:

____

____

6. Why is it important for email to be encrypted?

____

7. List six questions that should be asked during telephone screening.

____

____

____

____

8. Telephone documentation should include what seven pieces of information?

____

____

Scope of Practice Review

Indicate the calls described below that fall within the scope of practice for a medical assistant (MA) to respond to and the calls that should be directed to the provider (P).

Type of Call	Who Should Handle
Insurance questions	
Scheduling patient testing and clinic appointments	
Medical advice	
Requests for prescription refills	
Provider's family members	
General information about the practice	
Poor progress reports from a patient	
Requests for medications other than prescription refills	
Other providers	
Salespeople	
STAT reports	

Patient Confidentiality Activity

Because medical assistants must observe laws regarding both patient confidentiality and the patient's right to privacy, it is crucial for the medical assistant to understand and comply with legal and ethical principles and the restrictions governing issues of patient confidentiality. Indicate by marking the appropriate box whether the medical assistant may discuss a patient's medical condition or reveal details from the medical record.

	Yes	No	Yes, with Signed Release
Patient's spouse or family member			
Patient's employer			
Patient's attorney			
Another health care provider			
Patient's insurance carrier			
Referring provider's clinic			
Credit bureau or collection agency			
Member of the clinic staff, as necessary for patient care			
Other patient			
People outside the clinic (friends, acquaintances)			
Patient's parent or legal guardian, except concerning issues of birth control, abortion, or STDs			

CERTIFICATION REVIEW

These questions are designed to mimic the certification examination. Select the best response.

1. Telephone calls that may be handled by the medical assistant include all but which of the following?
   a. Billing questions
   b. Appointment changes
   c. Requests for prescription refills
   d. Calls from other providers

2. When a medical assistant is talking to a patient on the telephone and another line is ringing, what should the medical assistant do?
   a. Ask permission from the first caller to put her on hold, answer the second call and then ask permission from that caller to put him on hold, and go back to the first caller to finish up
   b. Put the first call on hold, answer the second call and handle that issue, then go back to the first caller
   c. Let the second line ring; it will be picked up by an answering system
   d. Finish with the first caller, then answer the second line
   e. Tell the caller, "Excuse me, I have another call I need to take"

3. Which of the following is *not* a good idea in a medical clinic?
   a. Using a speaker phone to listen to voice messages
   b. Speaking quietly on the telephone so patients at the clinic cannot hear
   c. Using a privacy screen to reduce the chance of being overheard on the telephone
   d. Using only email so you will not be overheard

4. Where should after-hours telephone messages be directed?
   a. The provider's home
   b. The medical manager's home
   c. A voice mail system or answering service/machine
   d. An email system
   e. The patient portal voice messaging system

5. Which of the following techniques should you follow when talking to older adult patients on the phone?
   a. If the patient is hearing impaired, speak slower, clearer, and a little louder
   b. Assume that they are senile or at least forgetful and repeat all the information several times
   c. If the person has difficulty understanding, simplify the information, ask if there are any questions, and try to explain patiently in simple terms
   d. A and c only

6. Which of the following are included as guidelines of the Health Insurance Portability and Accountability Act (HIPAA) for telephone communication?
   a. Determine if patients have specific instructions on who has been granted privilege to their private medical information
   b. Determine if patients have a particular number they want called for confidential communications
   c. Ask if it is acceptable to leave a message if patients are not at the number provided
   d. The medical assistant should identify himself or herself by name and say that he or she is an employee of the medical practice, using the complete official name of the practice
   e. All of the above

7. What is the best solution for handling a caller who refuses to give information after gentle prodding?
   a. Tell the patient to call back when he is ready to cooperate
   b. Hang up on the caller
   c. Take a message and then give it to the provider
   d. Argue with the patient, telling him that he is being unreasonable and that you need the information
8. What guideline should the administrative medical assistant follow when the phone rings?
   a. Answer by the end of the first ring if possible but definitely within three rings
   b. Answer after five rings
   c. Answer after two rings and before five rings
   d. Answer within a minute
   e. Let the call go to voice mail and answer/reply in the order it was received
9. What guideline should be followed before transferring a call to the appropriate party?
   a. Put the caller on hold, then transfer the call
   b. Put the caller on hold and contact the person to whom the call is going, to see if the person can speak to the caller
   c. Transfer the call immediately to free up additional lines
   d. Get the caller's full name, number, and any other situation-associated information
10. If a call is a medical emergency, what protocol should be followed in handling that type of situation?
    a. Make every attempt to obtain the caller's name and telephone number before assisting with making the 911 call if it appears the person is confused or unable to dial for himself or herself
    b. Prior to screening the call, direct the caller to call 911 if the caller believes he or she may be experiencing a life-threatening emergency
    c. Put the caller on hold and try to get the provider on the phone
    d. Tell the patient that you will call 911 and then call the patient back
    e. Both a and b

LEARNING APPLICATION

Critical Thinking

1. Answering the telephone professionally is critical in the health care profession. Meet with several classmates who each have written a scenario appropriate for an ambulatory care setting phone call. Now take turns being the caller and the medical assistant answering the clinic phone. Follow the steps outlined in Procedure 11-1 to cultivate your skills.

   ____

   ____

2. You are the medical assistant assigned to answering the telephone today. You receive a call from an angry patient. He wants to know why his bill was so high when he was only in the clinic with the provider for five minutes. What will happen if you become angry in retaliation? How should you handle this call in a professional manner?

   ____

   ____

   ____

3. Name four reasons why a potential patient will contact an ambulatory care facility by telephone.

____

____

____

4. Discuss the use of patient portal systems in your clinic. What are some advantages and disadvantages you should consider? What information might be addressed in a disclaimer related to use of patient portal systems?

Advantages:

a. _______________

____

b. _______________

c. _______________

d. _______________

e. _______________

f. _______________

g. _______________

Disadvantages:

a. _______________

____

b. _______________

____

c. _______________

d. _______________

____

5. Your clinic has just installed an automated telephone answering system. What steps might you take to aid your patients in understanding and using the system properly?

____

____

____

____

Case Studies

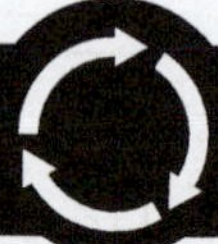

CASE STUDY 1

As Inner City Urgent Care continues to grow, increasing both patient load and staff, the existing telephone system, consisting of a simple intercom and four telephone lines, is no longer sufficient to handle the call volume and allow for full, immediate accessibility for all staff members. Callers are frustrated by the length of time it takes to get through and by long amounts of time spent on hold. Messages are often late in getting properly routed. Administrative medical assistant Karen Ritter, CMAA (NHA), suggests to clinic manager Jane O'Hara, CMA (AAMA), that an automated routing unit (ARU) might be more efficient for the growing clinic's needs. At the next regularly scheduled staff meeting, the provider-employers give the go-ahead to research an ARU.

CASE STUDY REVIEW QUESTIONS

1. ARU systems provide several options for callers that identify specific departments or services that callers can be connected with directly. What kinds of caller options might be appropriate for Inner City Urgent Care?

2. What can be done so the patient who has an emergency or who is hearing impaired can speak automatically to a live operator?

3. How can an ARU help staff members receive their calls more efficiently?

Role-Play Exercises

1. Effective telephone communication requires prompt and professional responses from medical assistants. With another student, role play the following scenarios as patient and as medical assistant. When you are finished role playing, write below what you said as the medical assistant.

   A. Patient Nora Fowler calls with a question about medication prescribed for her rheumatoid arthritis and insists on a call back from Dr. Mark King. Dr. King is presently on rounds at the hospital and will not be available until 4:30 PM. Nora's tone of voice indicates that she is upset, and she states that her medication is not helping her discomfort. It is clear from the conversation that Nora has discontinued taking her medication.

   B. While speaking on telephone line 1 with patient Bill Schwartz, who is calling to schedule a physical examination, medical assistant Nancy McFarland, RMA (AMT), receives another call on line 2 from a laboratory with a summary of emergency test results for another patient. Nancy knows that Dr. Ray Reynolds is waiting for the test results.

C. Medical assistant Ellen Armstrong, CMAS (AMT), takes a call from patient Juanita Hansen. Juanita is inquiring about a bill and indicating that her insurance carrier, Blue Cross, did not pay the entire fee for her son's last examination, which left her with a balance owed to Inner City Health Care. Clinic manager Marilyn Johnson, CMA (AAMA), is responsible for managing insurance claims and inquiries.

2. Team up with a classmate, one acting as the patient, the other as the medical assistant. Review the following scenario and the poor technique provided. Using the Attributes of Professionalism, take turns role-playing correct technique for the scenario, and write out the correct technique in the space provided.

SCENARIO: CALL FOR REFERRAL TO OTHER FACILITY

Herb Fowler needs to have a glucose tolerance test done at the laboratory next door and needs to make an appointment in your clinic for one week after the test is done. Role play placing the call to the patient.

Poor Technique

Medical Assistant: "Mr. Fowler, you need to call Johnston Labs to arrange for those tests. We'll see you after the tests are done."

Correct Technique

Hands-on Activities

1. Each morning, medical assistant Ellen Armstrong, CMAS (AMT), is responsible for transcribing messages left on the medical practice's answering machine the evening before. Using the message pad slips below, transcribe each message completely and appropriately. In the space for "Attachments," list any records, files, or documents that should be attached to the message slip for the recipient's review.

   A. "Ellen, this is Anna Preciado. Can you tell Marilyn Johnson, the clinic manager, that I won't be in tomorrow for the afternoon shift? I have a 101-degree temperature and bad flu symptoms. Check with Joe Guerrero to see if he can come in to sub for me as the clinical medical assistant. Yesterday he told me he would be available if I wasn't feeling well enough to come in. I know Dr. Lewis has several patients scheduled for clinical testing in the afternoon. I can be reached at 555-6622."

B. "This is Charles Williams. Dr. Lewis put me on a Holter monitor today. It's about 11:00 PM and one of the leads came off. I put it back on, but I am worried about whether I will have to do this test again. Can you call me tomorrow at home before 8:00 AM at 555-6124 or at the office after 9:00 AM at 555-8125? Thanks."

To:	Date: ___
From:	Time: ___
Telephone #:	
Message:	
	Initials:
Attachments:	

To:	Date: ___
From:	Time: ___
Telephone #:	
Message:	
	Initials:
Attachments:	

Research Activity

Jane Morgan has recently been diagnosed with amyotrophic lateral sclerosis (ALS). The patient is having difficulty getting to the second floor of her home, manual dexterity (buttons, dressing, bathing, eating), and driving to get to appointments. The patient lives alone at home. After today's visit with the doctor, you are asked to provide several local community resources to this patient for each of these issues. Research the available resources for a patient with this diagnosis and health-related difficulties and quality of life.

ATTRIBUTES OF PROFESSIONALISM

Discuss the following questions with another classmate or in a small group. During the discussion, consider how different people react in different ways, depending on their personalities, their patience, and their confidence levels. After the discussion, spend a moment in self-reflection to think of ways you can improve your telephone communication skills and how you would apply the Attributes of Professionalism, and write down your thoughts in your journal.

1. Have you ever conversed with someone on the telephone whom you could not understand? How would you apply the Attributes of Professionalism for communication?
2. Was the problem the language of the individual, or his or her accent, enunciation, or volume? How would you apply the Attributes of Professionalism for communication?
3. Would it have been easier to understand the individual if you were face-to-face with that person? How would you apply the Attributes of Professionalism for communication?

4. How did you handle the situation? Did you ask the person to speak louder, slower, or more clearly? How would you apply the Attributes of Professionalism for communication?
5. How do you think most people would handle a situation in which they could not hear the speaker clearly? What if the speaker were an older adult? A non–English speaker? A person in pain or very ill? How would you apply the Attributes of Professionalism for communication?

Name ______________________ Date __________ Score __________

CHAPTER 12

Patient Scheduling

VOCABULARY BUILDER

Misspelled Words

Find the words below that are misspelled; circle them, and correctly spell them in the spaces provided. Then insert the vocabulary terms from the list that best fit the scenarios below.

cluster scheduling	matrics	screaning
double booking	modified wave scheduling	stream scheduling
encription technology	practice-based scheduling	wave scheduling
______________	______________	______________

1. ______________ At Inner City Health Care, Ellen Armstrong, CMAS (AMT), schedules Mary O'Keefe for a 1:00 PM appointment for some blood work and Martin Gordon for a 1:00 PM appointment for a blood pressure check so Dr. King can assess whether his medication is at the proper level.

2. ______________ At Inner City Health Care, vaccinations are scheduled every 10 minutes from 10:00 AM to 12:20 PM on Mondays; Tuesday clinic hours are reserved for new patients only.

3. ______________ Three patients are scheduled to receive treatments in the first half hour of every hour.

4. ______________ Dr. Amy Cox prefers to see patients for regular gynecologic examinations in consecutive appointments scheduled from 8:30 AM to 11:30 AM and obstetric patients from 1:00 PM to 3:30 PM.

5. ______________ When patient Herb Fowler calls to set up an appointment with Dr. Winston Lewis for his chronic cough, Ellen Armstrong, CMAS (AMT), asks Herb a series of questions to ascertain the nature, extent, and urgency of his condition.

6. ______________ Dr. Winston Lewis prefers that each patient be assigned a specific time, scheduling at 30- or 60-minute intervals on a continuous basis throughout the day.

7. ______________________ An ophthalmologist schedules three patients at the beginning of each hour for comprehensive examinations, followed by single appointments every 10 to 20 minutes during the rest of the hour for quick, follow-up procedures such as removing eye patches or instilling eye drops.

8. ______________________ On the 15th day of each month, clinic manager Marilyn Johnson, CMA (AAMA), who is responsible for efficient patient flow at Inner City Health Care, asks each of the clinic's five providers to confirm their scheduling commitments for the upcoming month to block off unavailable times in the appointment book.

9. ______________________ The medical assistant uses software to protect patients' confidentiality in electronic format.

LEARNING REVIEW

Short Answer

1. Appointment books are legal documents recording patient flow. For a manual appointment system, where pencil is used for ease in rescheduling, what can the medical assistant do to ensure that a permanent record is secured?

____

____

____

2. For a computerized appointment system, what can a medical assistant do to ensure that a permanent record of patient flow is secured?

____

____

____

3. Name two primary goals in determining the best method for scheduling patient appointments.

____

____

4. What is the typical scheduling time for each of the following types of clinic visits for an internal medicine practice?

(1) New patient CPE ________

(2) Established patient routine follow-up ________

(3) Established patient CPE ________

(4) New patient sick ________

(5) Pap smear ________

(6) X-ray ________

5. What are six variables involved in the process of scheduling appointments for patients and other visitors to the ambulatory care setting?

____

____

____

____

6. Patient flow analysis sheets help medical practices determine the effectiveness of patient scheduling and devise plans for improving patient flow through the ambulatory care setting. What kinds of issues can a study of these data reveal?

7. What are the five steps of scheduling a specific appointment time for a patient?

8. Two ways of reminding patients of upcoming appointments are to give the appointment card personally to the patient and to mail the card to the patient. Identify a third reminder system. What procedures must be observed to protect patient confidentiality when using this third method?

9. Identify seven scheduling styles.

10. Identify the best scheduling system for the examples below, and explain the reasoning behind your choice.
    a. *Hospital emergency department.*
    b. *Laboratory for blood testing.*
    c. *Two or more patients need the same appointment time.*
    d. *Ambulatory care setting.*

CERTIFICATION REVIEW

These questions are designed to mimic the certification examination. Select the best response.

1. When should you schedule outpatient procedures?
   a. At the end of each day
   b. Best done with the patient present
   c. Easier with a calendar for visualization of days discussed
   d. Both b and c

2. What is the one principle above all else in scheduling for the clinic?
   a. Flexibility
   b. Neatness
   c. Accountability
   d. Estimation
   e. Open hours to accommodate early and late appointments

3. What, more than anything else, determines the success of a day in the ambulatory care setting?
   a. Patient care
   b. Efficient patient flow
   c. Operational functions
   d. Interpersonal skills

4. Which of the following are the types of scheduling systems?
   a. Wave, modified wave, double booking, mile-a-minute
   b. Open hours, wave, clustering, stream, double booking
   c. First-come, first-served; open hours; clustering
   d. Open hours, group appointments, wave-to-wave
   e. Modified cluster, stream to wave, open/closed hours

5. Below are guidelines to scheduling. Which one is correct?
   a. Urgent calls should be sent to the hospital, which is better equipped to handle them.
   b. Urgent calls should be screened or assessed before determining the best course of action.
   c. Referrals by other providers need to be seen immediately.
   d. Appointments for pharmaceutical and medical supply representatives should be referred to the provider.

6. Information that should be obtained from all new patients includes all but which of the following?
   a. The patient's full legal name
   b. The patient's birth date
   c. The patient's address and telephone numbers
   d. Reason for the visit
   e. The patient's family health history

7. Identify the term that refers to a current and accurate record of appointment times available.
   a. Schedule
   b. Screening
   c. Matrix
   d. Referral

8. What type of information is necessary for the patient to provide when scheduling his or her own procedure?
   a. Name of the provider ordering the procedure
   b. Name of patient's insurance information
   c. Social Security number and/or ID number
   d. The name of the procedure and preprocedure diagnosis
   e. All of the above

9. If there is going to be a delay by the provider of a half hour or longer to see the patient, what is the best course of action?
   a. Offer the patient the opportunity to run an errand, having them return at a specified time
   b. Offer to reschedule the appointment for another day, or later that day
   c. Offer the patient the opportunity to see another provider in the practice if available
   d. Any of the above

10. Which type of scheduling systems has major time-consuming problems seen at the beginning of the hour and minor problems seen from 20 minutes past the hour to half past the hour?
    a. Clustering
    b. Wave
    c. Modified wave
    d. Stream
    e. Open hours

LEARNING APPLICATION

Critical Thinking

1. Why is there no one best system of scheduling?

____

____

____

____

____

2. For the following situations, briefly explain which type of scheduling system you would choose and why.
   a. A four-provider practice has only two providers seeing patients at any one time. Three medical assistants share front- and back-office duties for all of the providers.
   b. An obstetrics practice specializes in high-risk pregnancies. There is one administrative and one clinical medical assistant.

____

____

____

____

3. With another person in your class, identify two or three public encounters where you have felt ignored or rushed as a customer. How does it make you feel? What suggestions would you make to the business to change that feeling?

____

____

____

____

____

____

Case Studies

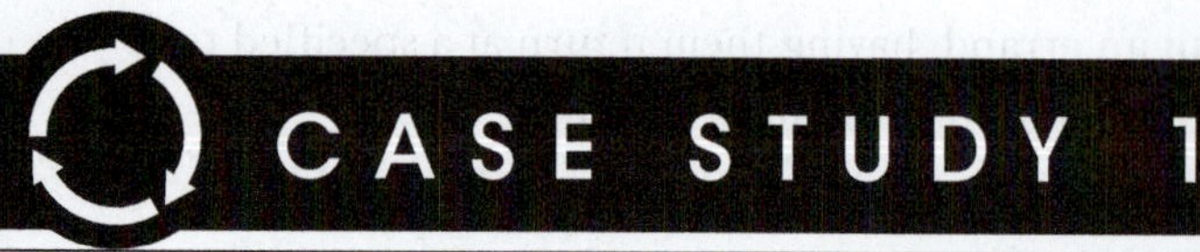

CASE STUDY 1

When patient Lenore McDonell falls from the examination table and lacerates her arm while attempting an independent transfer from the table to her wheelchair, clinical medical assistant Joe Guerrero, CMA (AAMA), alerts Dr. Winston Lewis, and the two begin to implement emergency procedures to control Lenore's bleeding and assess damage to the arm. Lenore's fall occurred at the end of her appointment, a routine checkup with Dr. Lewis.

Administrative medical assistant Ellen Armstrong, CMAS (AMT), must adjust Dr. Lewis's schedule to accommodate the emergency situation. Martin Gordon, a man in his mid-60s who has been diagnosed with prostate cancer, waits in the reception area for Dr. Lewis's next appointment. Martin's appointment, a 6-month follow-up, is expected to take 30 minutes. Martin is also being screened for depression related to his cancer diagnosis. Hope Smith, a new patient in good general health, is scheduled for a complete examination; she is due to arrive at Inner City Health Care within 20 minutes. Jim Marshall, an impatient and aggressive businessman, is scheduled for the first afternoon appointment after Dr. Lewis's lunch commitment. Mr. Marshall's appointment for a physical examination and ECG to investigate chest pains he has experienced recently is expected to take 45 minutes. Dr. Lewis's schedule is completely booked for the rest of the day.

CASE STUDY REVIEW QUESTIONS

1. What scheduling alternatives will Ellen offer Mr. Gordon, who is already waiting in the reception area? What special considerations regarding Mr. Gordon should Ellen take into account and why?

____

____

____

____

____

____

____

2. What is Ellen's first action regarding Ms. Smith, Dr. Lewis's next patient due to arrive? What scheduling alternatives should Ellen offer her?

____

____

____

____

____

3. What scheduling alternatives, if any, should Ellen present to Mr. Marshall? Explain your logic.

____

____

____

____

Hands-on Activity

Patient Martin Gordon has a 30-minute appointment scheduled with Dr. Lewis on Wednesday, February 7, 20XX for routine follow-up for prostate cancer. He calls the clinic on January 30 and would like to reschedule his appointment for two weeks later at 3:00 PM, the same time as his originally scheduled appointment. You mark through his name on the appointment schedule with a single line in red pen, and document the change in the patient's chart. Now, complete the appointment card below to be mailed to Mr. Gordon as a reminder of his new appointment time.

INNER CITY HEALTH CARE
8600 MAIN STREET, SUITE 200
RIVER CITY, XY 01234

Patient: ____________

has an appointment on

Mon. ___	at ___
Tues. ___	at ___
Wed. __________	at _______
Thurs. ___	at ___
Fri. ___	at ___

If unable to keep appointment, kindly give 24 hours' notice.

ATTRIBUTES OF PROFESSIONALISM

Patient scheduling is a vital part of the medical assistant's duties. How well you perform these duties will have an impact on patient care and is a reflection of the practice as a whole. Consider the Attributes of Professionalism and think about the following issues. Write in your journal how you react when you are the recipient, and how you would strive to display professional attributes when you are the one scheduling appointments for patients.

1. When you call a provider's clinic, do any of the following aggravate you? Do you think other people are aggravated by these? Determine an action that could alleviate all or some of the aggravation. Keep in mind that the situation might still exist (e.g., the receptionist might still have to ask a lot of questions), but how might he or she make the experience more pleasant?
   a. Being put on hold right away or too often
   b. The administrative medical assistant asking too many questions
   c. Not enough appointment time choices; that is, you have to wait too long for an appointment
   d. Not getting a real person; that is, having to listen to menu choices and make selections
   e. Other (add your own idea) ________________________________
2. When you visit a provider's clinic, do any of the following aggravate you? Determine an action that could alleviate all or some of the aggravation. Keep in mind that the solutions in this case are obvious and doable.
   a. The administrative medical assistant does not acknowledge you right away.
   b. The wait is too long.
   c. The waiting room is noisy, messy, or uncomfortable.
   d. There are no magazines of interest to you.
   e. Other (add your own idea) ________________________________.

Name ______________________________ Date __________ Score __________

CHAPTER 13

Medical Records Management

VOCABULARY BUILDER

Misspelled Words

Find the words below that are misspelled; circle them, and correctly spell them in the space provided. Then fill in the blanks in the following sentences with the appropriate terms. (Hint: Not all words will be used.)

accession record
caption
cross-reference
indexing
key unit
out-gide
perging
problem-orientated medical record
SOAP
source-orientated medical record
tickler file
unit

______________________ ______________________ ______________________

______________________ ______________________ ______________________

1. To remember to check with the reference laboratory on Friday to obtain patient Martin Gordon's test results, Ellen Armstrong, CMAS (AMT), places a note in her ______________________.
2. Every six months, Marilyn Johnson, CMA (AAMA), follows clinic policy and procedures for __________ inactive files to remove and archive those not in active use.
3. The organized method of identifying and separating items to be filed into small subunits is accomplished with the use of ______________________ units.
4. When Liz Corbin, CMA (AAMA), retrieves Annette Samuels's chart for Dr. Osborne, she places an ______________________ in the filing cabinet to show that the file has been removed from storage.
5. The ______________________ is a journal (or computer listing) where numbers in a numeric filing system are preassigned. The log sequentially lists numbers to be assigned to numeric records.
6. The file for Kent Memorial Hospital contains three indexing ______________________ to be considered when preparing the filing label.
7. If a ______________________ card is required in the alphabetic card file of a numeric filing system, such as when making note of an established patient's married name, a card is prepared that includes an *X* next to the file number to indicate that this card does not designate the primary location card for the file.

8. In the ______________________________ system of record-keeping, patient problems are identified by a number that corresponds to the charting relevant to that problem number; for example, asthma #1; dermatitis #2; and so on.

9. ______________________________ are used to identify major sections of file folders by more manageable subunits, such as GA–GE, or Miscellaneous. They are marked on the tabs of the guides.

10. Inner City Health Care uses the ______________________________ method of record-keeping, which groups information according to its origin—for example, laboratories, examinations, provider notes, consulting providers, and other types of information.

11. Some medical facilities have added variations of two additional letters, *E* and *R* or *I* and *E* to the ______________________________ approach, which stand for "Education for patient" and "Response of patient to education and care given" or "Implementation of the plan" (what was done) and "Evaluation, indicating whether care is effective, or results."

LEARNING REVIEW

Short Answer

1. Why is accurate, up-to-date, complete documentation in patient medical records essential in the ambulatory care setting?

2. Why is the POMR system commonly used by family practice clinics?

3. Why is a color-coding system effective in the ambulatory care setting?

4. How important is an effective, easy-to-use, and easy-to-access filing system to the efficiency of the ambulatory care setting?

5. List at least four advantages of EMR.

6. What does the acronym SOAPER stand for?

7. List three numeric filing systems that are used in medical facilities.

Indexing Units Exercise

Assign the correct units to the following items to be filed using the rule for filing patient records that is listed for each.

1. Names that are hyphenated are considered one unit.

   A. Jackson Hugh Levine-Dwyer

   unit 1 ____________ unit 2 ____________ unit 3 ____________

   B. Leslie Jane Poole-Petit

   unit 1 ____________ unit 2 ____________ unit 3 ____________

2. Seniority units are indexed as the last indexing unit.

   A. Keith Wildasin Sr.

   unit 1 ____________ unit 2 ____________ unit 3 ____________

   B. Gerald Maggart III

   unit 1 ____________ unit 2 ____________ unit 3 ____________

3. Titles are considered as separate indexing units. If the title appears with first and last names, the title is considered the last indexing unit.

   A. Dr. Louise Udolf

   unit 1 ____________ unit 2 ____________ unit 3 ____________

   B. Prof. Valerie Rajah

   unit 1 ____________ unit 2 ____________ unit 3 ____________

4. The names of individuals are assigned indexing units respectively: last name, first name, middle name, and succeeding names.

   A. Lindsay Adair Martin

   unit 1 ____________ unit 2 ____________ unit 3 ____________

   B. Abigail Sue Johnson

   unit 1 ____________ unit 2 ____________ unit 3 ____________

5. Foreign language units are indexed as one unit with the unit that follows. Spacing, punctuation, and capitalization are ignored.

   A. Joseph Jack dela Hoya

   unit 1 ____________ unit 2 ____________ unit 3 ____________

   B. Maurice John van de Veer

   unit 1 ____________ unit 2 ____________ unit 3 ____________

CERTIFICATION REVIEW

These questions are designed to mimic the certification examination. Select the best response.

1. What is the POMR also known as?

   a. A source-oriented medical record

   b. A SOAP/SOAPER system

   c. A traditional method

   d. A problem-oriented medical record

2. What best describes the SOAP/SOAPER format?
   a. A way to sanitize instruments
   b. A form of patient electronic records
   c. A type of filing system
   d. A specific charting system
   e. None of the above

3. If a patient needs to return for another examination in 6 months, you might use a reminder system. What is the name of that system?
   a. Reminder system
   b. Recall system
   c. Phone log
   d. Tickler system

4. What is the most common method of filing in today's medical clinic?
   a. Alphabetically
   b. Numerically
   c. By insurance
   d. By subject
   e. Color coding

5. If a medical document is filed in multiple places, what might be used to locate it?
   a. Index
   b. Out guide
   c. Cross-reference
   d. Multiple reference

6. What is the best method to use for making a correction in a paper medical record?
   a. Use a white-out product
   b. Scribble over the error with a magic marker
   c. Put *X*'s through the error
   d. Draw a single line through the error, make the correction, write *CORR* or *CORRECTION* above the area corrected, and add your initials and date
   e. Any of the above

7. What identifiable patient information should *not* appear on the outside of the chart?
   a. Patient's address
   b. Patient's Social Security number
   c. Patient's birth date
   d. All of the above

8. How long are closed files usually kept?
   a. 3 to 6 years beyond the statute of limitations
   b. 2 to 5 years
   c. Indefinitely
   d. 10 years
   e. 7 years unless kept on an EMR

9. Which of the following identifies the three types of cabinets used in medical clinics?
   a. Vertical, lateral, and movable
   b. Metal, hanging, and color coded
   c. Horizontal, lateral, and movable
   d. Open, locked, and movable

10. When are captions typically used?
   a. To separate file folders
   b. To identify major sections of file folders
   c. In vertical and lateral systems
   d. In color-coded and alpha-numeric systems
   e. A and c only

LEARNING APPLICATION

Filing Order Review

Using the numbers 1, 2, and 3, label the patient names in each group according to the correct filing order of names in an alphabetic filing system.

___ L. Sanders
___ Larry Paul Samuels
___ Lawrence P. Sanders

___ James Edward Reed Sr.
___ James Edward Reed
___ James Edward Reed Jr.

___ Lynn Elaine Brenner
___ Lynn Ellen Brenner
___ Lynn Eloise Brenner

___ Patrick Sam Saint
___ Patrick Sam St. Bartz
___ Paul Sam Saint

Critical Thinking

1. A patient's chart has been subpoenaed for pending malpractice litigation. In preparing the chart, you discover an error that was made when the results of the laboratory report were incorrectly documented in the chart. You have the original laboratory report. What should you do?

2. Research the statute of limitations in your state for medical records to determine how long a medical record should be kept. The statute will also tell you what triggers activity on a medical file that might dictate it be kept longer than normally indicated.

3. Identify the steps you might take in inspecting the charts before filing. What would you do if you found something missing or an unsigned report?

   a.

   b.

   c.

4. It has been said that filing records is the easiest task the medical assistant will perform, yet it is often the most difficult. What reasons can you give for this statement?

ATTRIBUTES OF PROFESSIONALISM

Records management is vital to the medical clinic. Imagine important test results missing or misfiled. How would not having accurate, up-to-date medical records for your patients impact their health care and also impact your job, professionally and legally?

Using several scenarios—for example, (1) missing PET scan and results to provider indicating a malignant tumor, (2) PT/INR lab report with out-of-range results not given to provider, and (3) breast biopsy filed/scanned to wrong patient chart—in your journal, write how each of these scenarios would impact the patient, provider, and practice. How would you apply the Attributes of Professionalism to make sure this type of error did not occur?

Would your answers be the same for paper and electronic records? If not, please explain.

Name ______________________________ Date __________ Score __________

CHAPTER 14

Written Communications

VOCABULARY BUILDER

Misspelled Words

Find the words below that are misspelled; circle them, and correctly spell them in the space provided. Then fill in the blanks in the passage below with the correct vocabulary terms. (Hint: Not all terms will be used.)

bond paper	modified block letter	proofread
form letter	optical character	simplified letter
full block letter	recognition	watermarque
keed	portfoleo	ZIP+4

_________________________ _________________________ _________________________

_________________________ _________________________ _________________________

There are four major types of letter styles in which medical assistants commonly write. Of these, the __________ style is the most time efficient because it does not use excessive tab indentations for the address, complimentary closure, or keyed signature. In the ______________ style, all lines begin at the left margin with the exception of the date line, complimentary closure, and keyed signature. Medical assistants may choose to use the ____________ style, which is the style of letter recommended by the Administrative Management Society. In this style, all lines are __________, or input by keystroke, flush with the left margin. When selecting paper supplies, the medical assistant should choose ______________ with a ____________, or image imprinted during the papermaking process that is visible when a sheet is held up to the light. When preparing letters for outgoing shipments, it is important for the medical assistant to pay attention to several factors, including addresses. Medical assistants should machine-print addresses (including the ____________ code) with a uniform left-hand margin so that the addresses can be read by the U.S. Postal Service's __________ __________ (OCR) software. One creative approach to letter composition is to create a ____________ or database of frequently used ________.

LEARNING REVIEW

Abbreviations Exercise

Write what each abbreviation stands for.

1. Enc. ______________________
2. c ______________________
3. P.S. ______________________
4. OCR ______________________
5. CAP ______________________
6. ROM ______________________
7. LC ______________________
8. WF ______________________

MATCHING

Match each common proofreader's mark to its meaning.

_____ 1. #		A. "Let it stand"
_____ 2. ^		B. Paragraph indent
_____ 3. BF		C. Insert space
_____ 4. STET		D. Move left
_____ 5.]		E. Italic type
_____ 6. [		F. Align type horizontally
_____ 7. :|		G. Insert
_____ 8. =		H. Boldface type
_____ 9. ITAL		I. Move right
_____ 10. ¶		J. Insert colon

Processing Mail Exercise

For each type of mail below, list the action the medical assistant should take or to what department or person the medical assistant should forward the mail.

Type of Mail	Action Taken
Invoices for supplies and equipment	
Magazines for reception area	
Insurance forms	
Patient payments	
Medical journals	
Personal or confidential letters	

CERTIFICATION REVIEW

These questions are designed to mimic the certification examination. Select the best response.

1. Which of the following represents the formal salutation?
   a. Signature of the sender
   b. Dear Mr. Marshal
   c. The return address of the sender
   d. The closing remark (such as "Sincerely")

2. When addressing an envelope, what is the proper way to list the state?
   a. Write out the state name completely
   b. Abbreviate the state name using at least the first four letters
   c. Use the official two-letter abbreviation and capitalize it
   d. Capitalize the first letter of the state name, followed by the second letter in lowercase
   e. Use any of the above so long as it is in uppercase letters and is written clearly

3. Which of the following would be incoming mail to a provider's clinic?
   a. Email
   b. Insurance forms
   c. Medical journals
   d. All of the above

4. The medical assistant may, with the provider's permission, sign which type of letters?
   a. The ordering of supplies or subscriptions
   b. Notification of collection procedures and reminder of payments
   c. Dismissal letters
   d. Consultation letters to a referring physician
   e. Only a and b

5. When addressing an envelope, which of the following is a true statement?
   a. The address should be machine-printed with a uniform left margin.
   b. All punctuation should be eliminated.
   c. Use dark ink on a light background and uppercase letters.
   d. All of the above

6. What types of envelopes are most often used in the medical clinic?
   a. Number 7
   b. Number 6¾
   c. Number 10
   d. Number 21
   e. Both b and c

7. In which type of letter format are the paragraphs indented five spaces?
   a. Simplified letter
   b. Unmodified block
   c. Indented modified block
   d. Standard modified block

8. What action is necessary before presenting any correspondence to the provider for signature?
   a. It should be date stamped.
   b. It must be checked for accuracy.
   c. It should be folded and put in an envelope.
   d. It must be typed on plain white paper.
   e. All of the above

9. What is the name of the computerized feature used when it is desirable to send the same letter, although personalized, to many different people?
   a. Word processing letters
   b. Mail merge
   c. Database letters
   d. Merge correspondence

10. What part of a letter includes the return address and perhaps a logo?
    a. Salutation
    b. Inside address
    c. Letterhead
    d. Reference heading
    e. Enclosure

LEARNING APPLICATION

Critical Thinking

1. With a group of classmates, organize a spelling bee of commonly misspelled medical words. Also include some nonmedical English words that are often misspelled. Conduct the spelling bee.

2. Practice composing business correspondence using all components. Procedure 14-1 is a helpful guide. Print a draft copy of your letter and use common proofreader's marks to indicate any corrections.

3. Rekey the above letter and practice folding it correctly. Procedure 14-3 provides step-by-step instructions.

4. Using a computer and printer, correctly address a number 10 envelope to a provider following all appropriate U.S. postal regulations. Print the envelope. Procedure 14-2 provides step-by-step instructions.

5. Once you have addressed your envelope, place your letter into the envelope correctly. Refer to Procedure 14-3 if you have forgotten how to insert the letter properly.

Case Studies

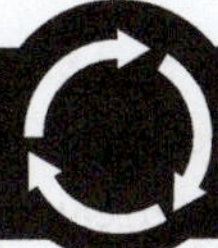

CASE STUDY 1

Ellen Armstrong, CMAS (AMT), enjoys working on correspondence for Inner City Health Care and takes pride in her written communication skills. As an ongoing project, clinic manager Marilyn Johnson, CMA (AAMA), asks Ellen to make suggestions for updating and revising the style manual used in the medical office for written communication guidelines. Ellen suggests the addition of a section in the style manual to discuss bias in language. Using bias-free language requires one to be sensitive when applying labels to individuals or groups and using sex-specific words and pronouns appropriately. For example, *dementia* is used instead of *crazy* or *senile.* Instead of using *layman,* consider using *layperson.* Apply *he* or *she* only in sex-specific usage. Marilyn and the provider-employer ask Ellen to implement the addition to the style manual.

CASE STUDY REVIEW QUESTIONS

1. Why is bias-free language an important consideration in written communication for the ambulatory care setting?

2. List other examples of biased language and give suggestions for bias-free alternatives.

Proofreading Exercise

Proofread the letter below, inserting the proper proofreader's marks directly onto the text to indicate how all errors should be corrected. (Consult your textbook for a list of common proofreader's marks and refer to a medical dictionary, if necessary.)

JAMES CARTER, MD, NEUROLOGY
Metropolitan University Medical Center, 8280 Wright Avenue, River City, XY 01234

February 2, 20XX

Mark King, M.D
Inner City Health Care
8600 Main Street, Suite 200
River City, XY 01234

RE: MARGARET THOMAS

Dear Dr. King:

Thank you for refering Margaret Thomas to my neurological practice. Margaret came to you recently as a new patient for a comprehensive physical examination to evaluate troubling symptoms she had been experiencing for several months. Margaret notices symtoms of tremor, difficulty walking, defective judgement, and hot flushes; she is not able to poinpoint the exacttime symptoms began. Your physical examination suggested the possible diagnoisis of parkingson's Disease. Margaret presented today for a complete nuerological evaluation.

MEDICAL/SURGICAL HISTORY. The patient is posiitive for the usual childhood diseases and the births of three children, following normal pregnancies. Her surgical history includes an Appendectomy performed 10 years ago. She has a food allergy to shellfish, but no known allergies to medications. She takes Pepto-Bismol and Metamusil for frequent stomach upset and constipation. She is a widow with two children, ages twenty three, twenty-five, and 29, and is a retired homemaker. She does not smoke and has an occassional glass of wine. Her family history is positive for colon cancer in her mother and parenteral grandfather and for lung cancer in her father.

PYHSICAL EXAMINATION. VITAL SIGNS: The patient has normal vital signs for a 52-year old Caucasian female. HEENT: The patient had a normacephalic and atraumatic exam. There is mild bobing of the head and facial expressions appear fixed. Pupils equal, round, react to light and acommodation. The fundi were benign. There was normal cup to disc ratio of 0.3. Tympanic Membranes were both clear and mobile. Her nose was clear, the oropharynz ws clear without any evidence of lezions. There was not cervical adenopathy, no thyromegely, or other masses. NECK: Musles of the neck are quite rigid and stiff. CHEST: Cear to percussion and auscultation. HEART: Regular rate and rhythm without murmurs or gallops, there was no jugular venous distention, no peripheral edema, no carotid buits. Pulses were 2+ and symetrical. ABDOMEN: Some what obese, but benigh. There was not organomegaly or masses. Bowel tones were normal. There was no rebound tenderness. BACK: Examination reveals loss of postural reflexe and patient stands with head bent forward and wals as if in danger of falling forward. There is difficulty in pivoting and loss of balance. GENITOURINARY: Normal. EXTREMITIES: Thre is moderate bradykinesia. Chracteristic slow, turning motion (pronationsupination) of the forearm and the hand, a motion of the thumb against the fingers as if rolling a pill between the fingers is noted. This condition seems to worsen when the patient is concentrating or feeling anxious.

NEUROLOGICAL. The patient was cooperative and answered all questions. There is no history past of mental disorders or cardiovascular disease. There is muscle weakness and rigidity in all four extremities. Intellect remains intact.

LABORATORY DATA: Urinanalysis reveals low levels of dopamin. Cat scan reveals degeneration of nerve cells occuring in the basel ganglia.

ASSESSMENT. Based on the patient history and neurologic examination, it appears most likely that the patient has mild to moderate Parkinsons Disease.

PLAN. 1. Recommend physical therapy focussed on learning how to manage difficult movements such as descneding stairs safely.
2. Exercises to maintain flexibility, motility, and mental well-being.
3. Levadopa to increase dopamine levels in the brain to control symptoms. Please advise the patient that alchohol consumption shoudl be limited because it acts antegonistically to levodopa.
4. Relaxation and stress management counseling.

PROGNOSIS. Parkinson's disease progresses slowly. Patient should be followed on a regular basis and observed for any signs of damentia which may result in about one-third of cases.

Sincerely,

James Carter, MD

DD: February 2, 20XX
DT: February 3, 20XX
JC/bl

ATTRIBUTES OF PROFESSIONALISM

Written communication is an essential component of professionalism. How well you communicate in writing, whether in correspondence or documenting in a patient chart or EMR, reflects on you and the medical practice.

Consider the Attributes of Professionalism and give an honest assessment of your skills.

1. How would you rate your written communication skills?
2. Are you able to express yourself accurately and concisely?
3. Are you able to communicate ideas effectively?

4. Is your spelling and punctuation accurate?
5. Are you capable of proofreading and editing for content?

In your journal, write how you would strive to improve your written communications to display the highest level of professionalism.

Name ______________________ Date ________ Score ________

CHAPTER 15

Medical Documents

VOCABULARY BUILDER

Misspelled Words

Find the words below that are misspelled; circle them, and correctly spell them in the spaces provided. Then insert the vocabulary terms from the list that best fit the descriptions below.

autapsy report	editor	progress notes
chart notes	electronic medical record	quality assurence
chief complaint	gross examination	review of systms
confidentiality agreement	history and physical examination	turnaround time
consultation report	outsourcing	voice recognition software
currant reports	patholigy report	
discharge summery	priveliged	

______________________ ______________________ ______________________

______________________ ______________________ ______________________

______________________ ______________________ ______________________

1. The part of the pathology report that describes the size and shape of a biopsy specimen is called a ______________________.

2. The part of patients' hospital records that describe their entire hospital stay, progress, and condition on release is called a ______________________.

3. The part of the patient's medical record that contains information related to the main reason for the encounter, as well as a synopsis of the patient's previous medical information, is called the ______________________.

4. Reports such as history and physical examinations that should be completed within 24 hours are called ______________________ reports.

5. Software that translates spoken sounds into written words is called ______________________.

6. A medical report generated to describe the examination of tissues or cells obtained through a surgical or medical procedure is the ______________________________ report.

7. The practice of contracting transcription with a service outside the clinic or hospital to a company where it can be done at a lower cost and with a faster turnaround time is called ______________________.

LEARNING REVIEW

Short Answer

1. List five personal attributes of the medical transcriptionist.

2. List at least four advantages of outsourcing.

3. Identify four ways the medical transcriptionist can be compliant with HIPAA.

4. Define the following types of medical documents.
   a. Chart notes (progress notes)
   b. History and physical examination (H and P) report:
   c. Radiology report:
   d. Operative report:
   e. Pathology report:

f. Consultation report:

___

___

g. Discharge summary:

___

h. Autopsy report:

___

___

5. Clinics using electronic medical records may delegate much of the medical transcriptionist's responsibility to other medical personnel. Identify the items below that may be entered into an electronic medical record by the medical assistant by writing *MA* next to the entry, and those items that must be entered by the provider as *P*.

Reason for the patient's visit ___

Chart notes ___

Vital signs ___

Transmitting a prescription to a pharmacy ___

Transmitting the medical record to another provider ___

Current medications ___

Entering the chief complaint ___

Abbreviations Exercise

Write what each abbreviation stands for.

1. EHR ___
2. MT ___
3. TAT ___
4. QA ___
5. VRS ___
6. CMT ___
7. CC ___
8. ROS ___
9. H and P ___
10. DS ___
11. OR ___
12. HIPAA ___

CERTIFICATION REVIEW

These questions are designed to mimic the certification examination. Select the best response.

1. The Association for Healthcare Documentation Integrity (AHDI) credentials which of the following?
   a. MTs
   b. CMTs
   c. CMTs and RMTs
   d. CMAs and RMAs

2. A digital dictation system allows you to measure to what length of time?
   a. The 30th or 90th of a minute
   b. 60 seconds
   c. The 10th or 100th of a minute
   d. 30 to 40 seconds
   e. 1⁄10 of a second

3. The medical report must have what elements?
   a. Correct date
   b. Signature or initials of the dictator
   c. Legible type
   d. All of the above

4. The specific time period in which a document is expected to be completed from the time it is received by the transcriptionist until it is returned to the provider and made part of the permanent medical record is called what?
   a. Filing time
   b. Turnaround time
   c. Completion time
   d. Return time
   e. Efficiency rating

5. What term applied to a radiology, pathology, or laboratory report usually indicates the need for immediate turnaround?
   a. ASAP
   b. Current
   c. Old
   d. STAT

6. Which of the following are included in the discharge summary?
   a. The reason for hospital admission
   b. The final diagnosis
   c. Follow-up instructions
   d. Description of what transpired while the patient was in the hospital
   e. All of the above

7. What does the abbreviation CMT stand for?
   a. Certified Medical Technician
   b. Certified Medical Transcriptionist
   c. Certified Medical Transcriber
   d. Certified Medical Technologist

8. A description of symptoms, problems, or conditions that brought the patient to the clinic is best described as what?
   a. Current medical issue
   b. Chief complaint
   c. Present problem
   d. Discharge summary
   e. Only b and c

9. Information that may be communicated only with the patient's permission or by court order is known as what?
   a. Privileged
   b. Private
   c. Confidential
   d. Disclosed

10. Gross and microscopic examinations may be performed on which of the following?
    a. Tissue samples
    b. Organs
    c. Body fluid removed during a surgical procedure
    d. Lesions
    e. All of the above

LEARNING APPLICATION

Critical Thinking

1. You have excellent keyboarding skills and understand word processing programs well. Your spelling and medical terminology skills, however, are poor. How will this impact your medical transcription productivity?

   ____

   ____

2. What could you do to improve your medical terminology and spelling?

   ____

   ____

   ____

3. List a minimum of three HIPAA confidentiality regulations that apply to medical transcription. What are the consequences of not being compliant?

   ____

   ____

   ____

4. Turnaround time is an important issue in medical transcription. What happens when the transcriptionist does not complete medical documents within the turnaround time limits? What steps could be taken to ensure compliance with turnaround time?

5. What if a serious error is made when transcribing a discharge summary and the court subpoenas the document because of litigation? What legal responsibility does the transcriptionist have for the accuracy of the document?

Case Studies

CASE STUDY 1

You are transcribing a report when you notice it is about your neighbor. The report states that the test run for multiple sclerosis is positive. You had just spoken to your neighbor yesterday and she was concerned that she hadn't heard from her provider and was wondering about the results of her tests.

CASE STUDY REVIEW QUESTIONS

1. What should you do?

Proofreading Exercise

Correct the following paragraph.

her past medical history is postivie for the usual childhood diseases and the births of to children following normal pregnancies. she has a negative past urgical history. she has no allergies To medications and takes tylenol for occasional headashes. She is married and has to children, ages 3 and 12 months. She does not smoke or drink.

ATTRIBUTES OF PROFESSIONALISM

While every task in the medical clinic requires professionalism, consider how the medical record and documentation contained in it require a high degree of accuracy. Thinking about your "competency" skills, describe in your journal how you would incorporate the required attributes of a medical transcriptionist. Consider your personality as it applies to this line of work. Are you comfortable working alone? Or do you prefer working in a more "social" environment?

Name ______________________ Date ________ Score ________

CHAPTER 16

Medical Insurance

VOCABULARY BUILDER

Misspelled Words

Find the words below that are misspelled; circle them, and correctly spell them in the spaces provided. Then insert the vocabulary terms from the list that best fit the descriptions below.

adjustmint	preautherization	resourse-based relative value scale
benefit period	prefered provider organization	self-insurance
Medicare Part D	primary care provider	usual, customarry, and reasonable
point-of-service plan	referral	

_______________ _______________ _______________

_______________ _______________ _______________

1. The _______________ is a doctor chosen by the patient who is the first doctor the patient sees and is responsible for making referrals for further treatment by a specialist or for hospitalization.
2. A _______________ allows the enrollee to have the freedom to obtain medical care from an HMO provider or to self-refer to a non-HMO provider at a greater cost.
3. The _______________ was developed using values for each medical and surgical procedure based on work, practice, and malpractice costs and factoring in regional differences.
4. _______________ is prior notice and approval that need to be obtained before services will be covered.
5. A _______________ is an organization of providers who network together to offer discounts to purchasers of health care insurance.
6. The _______________ is the specified time during which benefits will be paid under certain types of health insurance coverages.
7. The amount a provider writes off the patient's account is known as an _______________.
8. _______________ is prescription drug coverage by Medicare.

LEARNING REVIEW

Short Answer

1. What questions should the medical assistant ask when screening for medical insurance coverage?

2. What measures do managed care organizations employ to ensure cost-effective services?

3. List and describe the seven models of managed care organizations.

4. List seven pieces of information that should be maintained in a log regarding preauthorization, precertification, or referral procedures for various insurance carriers.

5. List and describe the three elements that should be considered when a provider's fee schedule is being created.

6. The insurance carrier generates an EOB and an RA. Explain what these are and who they are sent to.

7. List three examples of insurance fraud and three examples of insurance abuse.
   A. Fraud:

   B: Abuse:

8. Discuss the importance of Workers' Compensation insurance.

Matching

Match the statements below to the appropriate Medicare part.

_________	1. Covers outpatient expenses including providers' fees, lab tests, and radiologic studies	A. Medicare Part A
_________	2. Covers hospital admission and stays	B. Medicare Part B
_________	3. Offers prescription drug coverage for everyone covered by Medicare	C. Medicare Part C
_________	4. Referred to as Medicare advantage plans	D. Medicare Part D
_________	5. Does not require a monthly premium	
_________	6. Has a "donut hole" or coverage gap	
_________	7. Will start paying for services after a $204 deductible has been met	
_________	8. Requires a monthly premium	
_________	9. Covers hospice care	
_________	10. Covers charges for durable medical equipment	

CERTIFICATION REVIEW

These questions are designed to mimic the certification examination. Select the best response.

1. What is the portion of the medical fees that the patient needs to pay at the time of services called?
   a. Co-payment
   b. Fee for service
   c. Out-of-pocket expenses
   d. Premium

2. Which of the following is the largest medical insurance program in the United States?
   a. Blue Cross/Blue Shield
   b. Medicaid
   c. Medicare
   d. TRICARE
   e. ACA (Obamacare)

3. What is the cost that patients must pay each month (sometimes provided by their employers) called?
   a. Out-of-pocket expense
   b. Co-payment
   c. Premium
   d. Relative value scale

4. Which of the following describes HIPAA?
   a. It is about confidentiality, patient privacy, and the security of personal health information.
   b. It protects health insurance coverage for workers and their families when they change or lose their jobs.
   c. It includes national standards for electronic health care transactions.
   d. It establishes rules for national identifiers for providers, health plans, and employers.
   e. Only a and c

5. Time-dependent limitation of coverage is known as what?
   a. Nonallowed service
   b. Exclusion
   c. Out-of-pocket service
   d. Expensive service

6. Which term best describes a statement summarizing how the insurance carrier determined reimbursement for services and is received by the patient?
   a. Explanation of benefits (EOB)
   b. Remittance advice (RA)
   c. Day sheet
   d. Personal financial statement
   e. Monthly provider statement

7. What is the medical insurance that was designed to assist those on public assistance, low-income persons over the age of 65, people with disabilities between the ages of 18 and 65, and those that are blind called?
   a. Medicare
   b. CHAMPUS
   c. TRICARE
   d. Medicaid

8. What step(s) should the medical assistant take to ensure that there is a flow of adequate income in the clinic or office?
   a. Bill the insurance carrier promptly
   b. Complete claim forms properly
   c. Keep track of aging accounts
   d. Bill patients as needed
   e. All of the above

9. What are improper billing practices considered?
   a. Fraud
   b. Nonproductive
   c. Abuse
   d. Risky

10. The person covered under the terms of an insurance policy is called what?
    a. Primary
    b. Secondary
    c. Beneficiary
    d. Elector
    e. None of the above

LEARNING APPLICATION

Critical Thinking

1. When children of married parents are covered under both parents' policies, how is the birthday rule used to determine which policy is primary?

2. You are the medical assistant working the front desk and one of your responsibilities is to screen patients for insurance. What questions will you ask when collecting these data, and how will you word each question so that accurate information is received from the patient?

3. An established patient is seen today by the provider, who determines that a liver scan is necessary to determine a diagnosis. You must ascertain if this procedure is a covered benefit, determine what the payment rate will be by the carrier, and secure preapproval if necessary. How will you go about collecting this information?

4. You must establish proof of eligibility for a patient with Medicaid. How will you go about doing this?

5. Do you agree with the policy that managed care may set limits on services or length of services? Why or why not? Give your rationale.

Case Studies

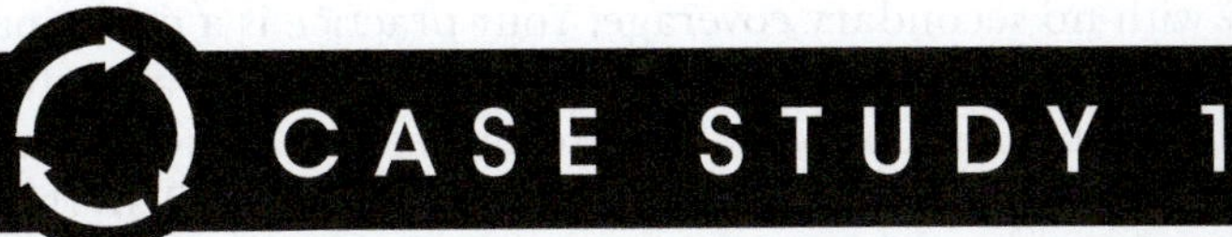

Lourdes Austen, a 1-year survivor of breast cancer, is covered by an HMO. Lourdes's primary care provider, Dr. King, recommends that Lourdes receive a colonoscopy because she has a family history that is positive for colon cancer, and medical studies have demonstrated a link between colon and breast cancers in families. Lourdes's HMO requires preauthorization before a specialist's care can be provided. Dr. King supplies the referral to the gastroenterologist who will perform the colon screening test and gives Lourdes the necessary completed referral form to take with her to her scheduled appointment. During the colonoscopy procedure, one benign polyp is removed, and the gastroenterologist requests that Lourdes return for a follow-up examination in 1 week.

Lourdes makes an appointment with the specialist's administrative medical assistant. When she returns 1 week later, the medical assistant informs Lourdes that she must have a new referral form for the clinic visit or the HMO will not approve payment; Lourdes will have to pay for the examination herself. "But we drove 40 minutes to get here, and no one ever told me I'd need another form for this. I thought it was all covered under the colonoscopy," Lourdes says.

CASE STUDY REVIEW QUESTIONS

1. Lourdes's HMO policy requires preauthorization. Is there anything that can be done to secure a proper referral without having to schedule another appointment for the patient or force the patient to pay for the clinic visit?

____

____

____

____

2. What is the role of the specialist's administrative medical assistant in this situation? Could the situation have been prevented?

____

____

____

____

Hands-On Activities

1. **Obtaining a Referral for a Patient.** Divide the class into pairs. One student in each pair will assume the role of the medical assistant, while the other assumes the role of a representative at the insurance company. The medical assistant will ask the insurance representative the following questions to help students understand the important duty of obtaining a referral for a patient:
   a. Is the service/procedure covered by the insurance? (If so, the medical assistant must provide the DOS at this time to indicate when the initial service will potentially take place.)
   b. Referral/authorization number.
   c. Co-payment amount and deductible information.
   d. How many visits are authorized?
   e. What is the expiration date?
   f. Name and telephone number of the contact person (or the person with whom you spoke).

2. **Calculating Allowed Charges and Determining Patient Responsibility.** A new patient, Carol Cooper, age 67, has just received services at the family practice clinic where you work. Her charges for the day come to $200.00. She is a Medicare beneficiary with no secondary coverage. Your practice is a participating provider with Medicare and accepts assignment, which allows $100.00 for the service. You have already contacted Medicare and verified that her Medicare deductible responsibility has already been met, and that her services are covered. It is now time to calculate what Medicare will potentially pay for her services. Fill in the appropriate amounts.

   a. New patient clinic visit charge: ______

   b. Allowed amount for the service according to Medicare's fee schedule: ______

      1. 80% to be paid by Medicare: ______

      2. Amount to be written off by the provider: ______

      3. Patient responsibility: ______

ATTRIBUTES OF PROFESSIONALISM

You might be asking yourself, "What does professionalism have to do with medical insurance?" Think back to each of the Attributes of Professionalism and write in your journal how your knowledge and actions affect the patient and the medical clinic. For example, consider the patient that does not have insurance, but is in urgent need of medical care. Describe actions you would take in a professional manner to assist that patient. If your responsibility includes asking patients for money (e.g., co-payments, balance on account, fees that are required to be paid up front), how will you use the Attributes of Professionalism in your communication, presentation, competency, initiative, and integrity? You may use the above example, or any other example related to medical insurance, to reflect upon professionalism.

____

____

____

____

____

____

Name ______________________ Date ________ Score ________

CHAPTER 17

Medical Coding

VOCABULARY BUILDER

Misspelled Words

Find the words below that are misspelled; circle them, and then correctly spell them in the spaces provided.

bundeled codes
claim register
Current Procedural Terminoligy
encounter form
explanation of benifts
Healthcare Common Procedure Coding System
International Classification of Deseases
modifyers
point-of-service device
Uniform Bill 04 (UB-04)

_______________ _______________ _______________

_______________ _______________ _______________

Definitions

Write the definitions of the following terms or phrases.

1. Bundled codes
____
2. Claim register
____
____
3. Current Procedural Terminology (CPT)
____
____
4. Encounter form
____
____
____

5. Explanation of benefits

6. Healthcare Common Procedure Coding System (HCPCS)

7. *International Classification of Diseases*, 10th Revision, Clinical Modifications (ICD-10-CM)

8. Point-of-service (POS) device

9. Uniform Bill 04 (UB-04)

10. Modifier

LEARNING REVIEW

Short Answer

1. CPT is updated annually and published by the American Medical Association. It is divided into six main sections. List them in the order in which they appear in the CPT codebook.

2. What are the steps to be taken to locate an ICD-10-CM code?

3. Errors in coding insurance claims can have far-reaching effects for both the patient and the provider. Name three effects.

4. Differentiate between bundled and unbundled codes.

5. List five common errors (and how to void those errors) that may occur when completing insurance claim forms.

6. Identify seven basic elements necessary to have documented in a compliance program.

Diagnosis and Procedure Identification

For each entry in the following table, insert a D for diagnosis or a P for procedure on the first line. Then, enter the appropriate diagnosis or procedure code, referencing the textbook, the current revision of the ICD, or the current edition of the CPT.

Diagnosis/Procedure	Entry	Code
	1. Supplies and materials provided by the physician over and above those usually included with the office visit	
	2. Poisoning by unspecified drugs, medication and biologic substances, undetermined, initial encounter	
	3. Anorexia nervosa, binge eating/purging type	
	4. Pneumonocentesis, puncture of lung for aspiration	
	5. Other specified diabetes mellitus with ketoacidosis without coma	
	6. Urinalysis, microscopic only	
	7. Sleep related bruxism	
	8. Pneumocystosis	
	9. Amniocentesis, diagnostic	
	10. Infectious mononucleosis, unspecified without complication	
	11. Gait training (includes stair climbing)	
	12. Medical testimony	
	13. Therapeutic, prophylactic, or diagnostic injection (specify substance or drug); subcutaneous or intramuscular	
	14. Newborn affected by maternal use of other drugs of addiction	

Research Activity

What is medical necessity? Using the Internet, research the definition of medical necessity and cite several examples.

CERTIFICATION REVIEW

These questions are designed to mimic the certification examination. Select the best response.

1. A provider's fee profile reflects which of the following?
   a. An average of all the practice's fees
   b. The amount of each charge for each service; can affect the provider's reimbursement for those services
   c. An average of fees charged over a period of 3 months
   d. The amount paid by insurance carriers

2. A diagnosis code of R30.0 has been entered on the claim form. What system is used to assign that code?
   a. CPT
   b. ICD-9-CM
   c. ICD-10-CM
   d. HCPCS
   e. RVS

3. In the CPT manual, the description of the level of E&M codes includes which of the following?
   a. Complexity of the medical decision making
   b. Level of history taken
   c. New versus established patient
   d. All of the above

4. What type of confirming will the insurance claims processor perform?
   a. There are no exclusions or restrictions for payment of that diagnosis.
   b. The provider has contracted with the insurance carrier.
   c. The procedure relating to the diagnosis is medically necessary.
   d. Must know who the claim is from.
   e. All of the above

5. Deliberately billing a higher rate than appropriate for the procedure that was performed to obtain greater reimbursement is known as what?
   a. Encoding
   b. Down-coding
   c. Up-coding
   d. Exploding

6. What is the best way to prevent a breach of confidentiality when processing insurance claim forms?
   a. Ask the patient, parent, or guardian to sign an authorization to release medical information form before the claim is completed
   b. Ask the patient for verbal approval before sending in the claim
   c. Have the patient write a letter requesting that the information be forwarded
   d. Have the insurance carrier contact the patient
   e. Have the provider note the approval in the chart note of the visit

7. When coding, which of the following is considered imperative?
   a. To be as precise as possible
   b. Not to guess
   c. Not to code what is not there
   d. All of the above

8. Which of the following would be considered a benefit of submitting claims electronically?
   a. Improves cash flow
   b. Ensures consistency
   c. Reduces the amount of supplies required
   d. Reduces errors
   e. All of the above

9. Using an electronic device for direct communication between medical offices and a health care plan's computers is called what?
   a. Subrogation
   b. Point-of-service
   c. Diagnosis-related groups
   d. Prospective payment

10. What is the most common claim form in the ambulatory setting?
    a. CMS-1450
    b. HCFA-1000
    c. CMS-1500
    d. CPT-1500
    e. HCPCS-04

LEARNING APPLICATION

Critical Thinking

1. Electronic claims filing is mandatory for Medicare. Karen recently graduated from an accredited medical assisting program and is employed in the insurance department of a busy medical practice. She has asked her supervisor how she can gain more knowledge in coding and electronic billing procedures and how she might decrease the number of rejected claims. How would you respond if you were the supervisor?

____

____

____

____

____

____

2. The supervisor has given Karen a number of rejected claims and asks her to determine why the claims were denied and to maintain a log of these reasons to be discussed at the next staff meeting. How should Karen proceed with this assignment?

____

____

____

3. Karen finds that many claim forms were rejected because important information was omitted. How might Karen suggest corrections for these omissions?

____

____

____

Case Studies

CASE STUDY 1

Lourdes's colonoscopy required the following diagnoses and procedures. Using the appropriate coding manuals, give the correct coding for processing the insurance claim for this patient.

CASE STUDY REVIEW QUESTION

Colonoscopy, flexible, proximal to splenic flexure; with biopsy, single or multiple _____

Benign neoplasm of the colon, unspecified _____

Family history of malignant neoplasm of digestive organs _____

Personal history of malignant neoplasm of the breast _____

Office or other outpatient visit of an established patient requiring 2 of 3 key components (low to moderate severity), physician typically spends 15 minutes face-to-face with patient or family _____

CPT Review

For each procedure listed, give the correct procedure code and name the CPT section in which the code can be found.

Chemotherapy administration, intravenous infusion technique, up to 1 hour _____ _______________

Hepatitis B surface antibody (HBsAb) _____ _______________

Simple repair of superficial wounds of scalp, neck, axillae, external genitalia, trunk, or extremities (including hands and feet) 7.6 to 12.5 cm _____ _______________

Electrocardiogram, routine ECG with 12 leads; with interpretation and reports _____ _______________

Hepatic venography, wedged or free, with hemodynamic evaluation, radiologic supervision and interpretation _____ _______________

Hepatitis Be antigen (HBeAg) _____ _______________

Anesthesia for arthroscopic procedures of hip joint _____ _______________

ATTRIBUTES OF PROFESSIONALISM

Have you considered whether you would like to be an insurance coder and biller? Which of the Attributes of Professionalism would be most valuable to an insurance biller and coder? Consider the requirements of the position and write in your journal why you would be a good coder and biller (or not). Which Attributes of Professionalism best describe you and would be most helpful in that role?

Name ______________________ Date __________ Score __________

CHAPTER **18**

Daily Financial Practices

VOCABULARY BUILDER

Misspelled Words

Find the words below that are misspelled; circle them, and correctly spell them in the spaces provided. Then insert vocabulary terms from the list that best fit into the descriptive sentence below.

accounts payible	day sheat	payee
accounts recievable	debit	pegboard system
adjustments	encounter form	petty cash
balance	guaranter	poasting
cashier's check	leadger	voucher check
certified check	money market savings account	
credit	notary	

______________________ ______________________ ______________________

______________________ ______________________ ______________________

1. ______________________ A record of daily patient transactions used in conjunction with pegboard systems
2. ______________________ Money (small amount of cash) kept in the clinic for minor or unexpected expenses such as postage-due mail or coffee supplies
3. ______________________ Column to the right of the debit column used for entering payments; decreases the balance due by reducing the amount in the debit column.
4. ______________________ As a noun, this term denotes the amount owed; as a verb, the term means to record the difference between the debit and credit columns and show any amount due
5. ______________________ Accounting function that describes the act of recording financial transactions in bookkeeping or accounting systems
6. ______________________ Indicate any insurance payment, personal discount or write-off, or any other subtraction for the amount that needs to be recorded

7. ______________________ Sum owed by a business for services or goods received (bills, refunds or overpayments, replenishment of petty cash, etc.)

8. ______________________ Total amount of money owed to a business for services or goods supplied

LEARNING REVIEW

Short Answer

1. Identify six habits essential to creating and maintaining accurate paper financial records.

2. Identify seven of the nine features that may be part of a checking account.

3. What are five rules to ensure that checks are properly written and recorded?

4. Give three reasons why it is important to ensure that proper control is utilized when purchasing supplies and equipment.

5. When office supplies arrive, what should be done to verify that the correct items and quantities have been received? What should be done to prepare the invoice for payment?

6. Describe the following types of checks, which are different from checks issued from a standard business checking account.

   (a) Cashier's check

   (b) Certified check

(c) Money order

(d) Voucher check

(e) Electronic check

7. Adjustments are entries made to a patient's account. Name three reasons why adjustments may sometimes be made to a patient's account.

8. Deposits are generally made daily. All checks to be deposited must be endorsed. Define *endorsement.* Identify the best method of endorsing checks in the clinic setting and describe the benefits of using this method.

9. If a check is returned to the ambulatory care setting for nonsufficient funds (NSF), what procedures should be followed?

10. It is crucial to balance all financial information for each day and for the month's end. Month-end figures on the day sheet must agree with the patient ledgers. Why is it important to go through this time-consuming accounting process?

11. Differentiate between bookkeeping and accounting.

12. How should a medical clinic establish and maintain a petty cash system?

____

____

____

____

____

____

____

____

CERTIFICATION REVIEW

These questions are designed to mimic the certification examination. Select the best response.

1. What is the pegboard system of bookkeeping sometimes called?
   a. Write-it-once system
   b. Ledger system
   c. Double-entry system
   d. Duplicated page system

2. What does the acronym *NSF* stand for?
   a. Nonsufficient funds
   b. Not sufficient funds
   c. Not satisfactory funding
   d. Negligent status of funding
   e. None of the above

3. What is the purpose of a restrictive endorsement stamp?
   a. Stamp on the ledger to signify that payment has been made
   b. Stamp the doctor's signature on insurance forms and other documents
   c. Stamp on the statement to signify that you have sent a check
   d. Stamp on the back of a check to signify "for deposit only"

4. What best describes reconciling a bank statement?
   a. Reconciling should be done every month
   b. The checkbook entries should be checked against the bank statement
   c. The reconciling should be done daily by computer
   d. All reconciling should be done in ink to avoid any unauthorized entries
   e. Both a and b

5. If a check has been deposited and is now returned because of nonsufficient funds, what is the first step to take?
   a. Redeposit the check
   b. Call the bank that returned it and verify availability of funds so the check can then be redeposited
   c. Call the patient who wrote the check
   d. Discard the check and credit the amount back to the patient's account

6. The pegboard system consists of which of the following?
   a. Day sheets
   b. Ledger cards
   c. Encounter forms
   d. Receipt forms
   e. All of the above

7. What is the most common method of tracking a patient's balance?
   a. The pegboard system
   b. Computerized financial systems
   c. The ledger card
   d. Both a and b

8. In cases of divorced parents and blended families, what is the parent with physical custody of the child, considered the one responsible for payment if the child is not insured with a contracted insurance carrier, referred to as?
   a. The payee
   b. The guarantor
   c. The subscriber
   d. Custodian of records
   e. None of the above

9. Who is the Advanced Beneficiary Notification form used primarily for?
   a. Medicaid patients
   b. HMO patients
   c. Medicare patients
   d. CHAMPUS patients

10. Which of the following is another name for the patient encounter form?
    a. Charge slip
    b. Superbill
    c. Pegboard form
    d. Procedure form
    e. Both a and b

LEARNING APPLICATION

Critical Thinking

1. Discuss the types of checks identified in the text. Give an example of how each might be used or seen in the ambulatory care medical setting.

____

____

____

____

____

2. Check with a local bank or two to determine how after-hours deposits are made. Are any special supplies necessary? What is the bank's responsibility? What is the responsibility of the office staff?

____

____

____

____

____

____

____

3. When you reconcile the practice's bank statement, you see that a check written almost 30 days ago to one of your suppliers has not been deposited. What course of action do you take, if any?

____

____

____

____

4. Even when a computer software system is used for the management of the practice's finances, discuss why following the bookkeeping guidelines for a manual system still has merit.

____

____

____

____

Hands-on Activities

1. Administrative medical assistant Ellen Armstrong, CMAS (AMT), is responsible for assisting the clinic manager and accountant in performing accounts payable activities for Inner City Health Care. On September 4, she receives a $323.45 bill from RJ Medical Supply Company for blood pressure equipment the office received on August 30. Noting that the company demands payment within 30 days of billing, Ellen writes a check disbursing funds to the company on September 15. The balance in the clinic's checking account before this check is written is $26,100.00. Using this information, write out the check and stub below. Ellen will submit the check to Angie Osborne, M.D. for her signature.

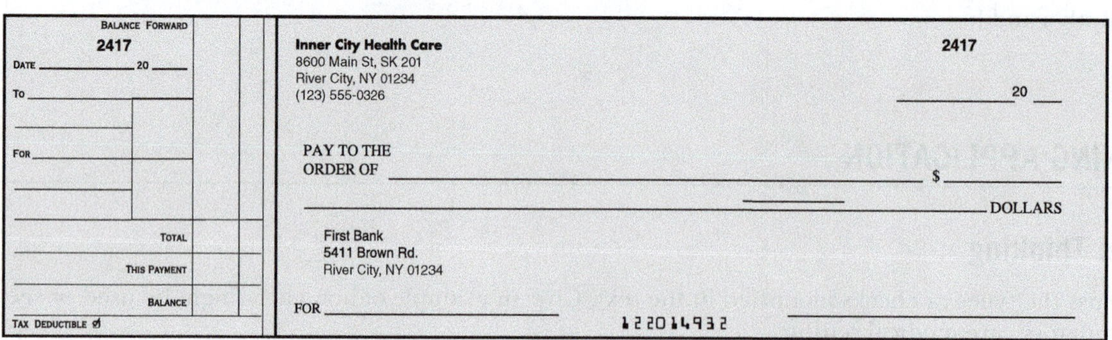
BALANCE FORWARD
2417
DATE __________ 20 ____
To __________
FOR __________
TOTAL
THIS PAYMENT
BALANCE
TAX DEDUCTIBLE ☐

Inner City Health Care
8600 Main St, SK 201
River City, NY 01234
(123) 555-0326

2417

__________ 20 ____

PAY TO THE ORDER OF __________ $ __________

__________ DOLLARS

First Bank
5411 Brown Rd.
River City, NY 01234

FOR __________

122014932

2. Clinic manager Marilyn Johnson, CMA (AAMA), is responsible for purchasing office supplies for Inner City Health Care. On September 10, Marilyn completes purchase order #1742 to Mayflower Supply, requested by administrative medical assistant Ellen Armstrong. The items are taxed at 8%, and the shipping fee is prepaid. The items are billed and shipped to Inner City Health Care; the terms are net due 30 days. Complete the purchase order form below.

PURCHASE ORDER **NO. 1742**

Bill To:	Ship To:	Vendor:

REQ BY	BUYER	TERMS

QTY	ITEM	UNITS	DESCRIPTION	UNIT PR	TOTAL
				SUBTOTAL	
				TAX	
				FREIGHT	
				BAL DUE	

Inner City Health Care
8600 Main Street, Suite 201
River City, NY 01234
(123) 555-0326

Mayflower Supply, Inc.
642 East 65th Street
River City, NY 01234
(123) 555-9999

2 boxes of fax paper, #62145, at $8.99 a box

5 day-view desk calendars, #24598, at $4.25 each

4 cases of copier paper, #72148, at $20.00 a case

5 boxes of highlighter pens, 12 to a box, #26773, at $3.98 a box

4 computer printer cartridges, #96187, at $49.99 each

ATTRIBUTES OF PROFESSIONALISM

The financial health of the medical clinic depends upon accurate, timely, and sound financial practices. Although you may determine a career in the clinical side of medical assisting is more to your liking, you must be aware of and excel in all aspects of the clinic's activities. Thinking about responsibilities related to the clinic's financial practices, how would you incorporate your skills and knowledge in this area with the Attributes of Professionalism? Do you keep personal financial records? Do you balance your checkbook and reconcile your bank statements at least monthly? Consider at least two clinic scenarios (such as being designated to balance the daily co-payments and updating the accounts receivable and payables for your month-end provider meeting) and write in your journal how you would accomplish these tasks, incorporating the Attributes of Professionalism.

Name ______________________ Date ________ Score ________

CHAPTER **19**

Billing and Collections

VOCABULARY BUILDER

Misspelled Words

Find the words below that are misspelled; circle them, and correctly spell them in the spaces provided. Then match each vocabulary term to its definition below.

accounts recievable ratio	Fair Debt Collection Practice Act	statute of limatations
collection ratio	probate court	Truth-in-Lending Act
____________	____________	____________

1. ____________ Also known as the Consumer Protection Act of 1967; an act requiring providers of installment credit to state the charges in writing and to express the interest as an annual rate
2. ____________ Debt collectors are not allowed to use their positions to collect a debt using any manner of work performance that is found to be abusive, deceptive, or unethical
3. ____________ Defines the period of time in which legal action can take place
4. ____________ A method used to gauge the effectiveness of the clinic's billing practices; shows the status of collections and the possible losses in the medical facility
5. ____________ Measures the speed with which outstanding accounts are paid

LEARNING REVIEW

Short Answer

1. A billing efficiency report allows for careful monitoring of follow-up bills; that is, whether they were paid, if the insurance has paid, and an assessment of the patient's responsibility for payment. What five pieces of data are included in these reports from which production efficiency is calculated?

2. Describe the importance of the Truth-in-Lending Act as it relates to a medical clinic.

3. Identify and explain the five most common reasons some patient accounts become past due.

4. In the pegboard system, what method is used to identify the age of accounts?

5. Aging accounts using computer software is simple. Name five account aging criteria which the computer program can perform.

6. The computer can also generate accounts receivable reports. Name three pieces of information included on a computer-generated accounts receivable report.

7. Collection agencies generally provide two services to an ambulatory care facility. Name and describe each type of service.

8. Collection of fees when a patient has died is directed to the executor of the estate. Place an *X* next to each action below that represents a responsible action in collecting past due accounts from deceased patients' estates.

_	If there is no known administrator, address the statement to "Estate of [insert patient's name]" and mail to the patient's last known address
_	Send an invoice via certified mail with a complete breakdown of all monies owed to the deceased patient's spouse or closest relative, noting that the survivor is responsible for making payment in full
_	Mail the account information via certified mail, return receipt, to the administrator of the estate, whose name can be obtained from the probate department of superior court
_	If unsure how to proceed, contact the clinic's attorney or the probate court for advice

9. With regard to collections, the statute of limitations is usually defined by the class of the overdue account. Name the three classes of accounts.

____

____

10. There are certain legal rules and ethical guidelines to follow when placing collection calls. Circle all that apply.
    a. Callers must identify themselves and ascertain that the person they are talking to is the responsible party.
    b. Threaten to turn the account over to a collection agency.
    c. If you make contact with the debtor's place of business, do not reveal to any third party the nature of the call.
    d. Do not make repeated calls to the debtor's friends or family.

CERTIFICATION REVIEW

These questions are designed to mimic the certification examination. Select the best response.

1. What is the term for patients who owe money but have moved and left no forwarding address?
    a. Deadbeats
    b. Skips
    c. Nonpayers
    d. Dead accounts

2. Statutes of limitations vary from state to state but should be investigated if an unpaid account is more than how old?
    a. 1 year
    b. 3 years
    c. 5 years
    d. 10 years
    e. There is no time limit if the account is more than a certain amount

3. Lack of payment from a patient may not be considered serious until after how long?
    a. 30 days
    b. 60 days
    c. 90 days
    d. 120 days

4. What should the medical assistant do for an insurance claim pending more than 45 days?
   a. Call the carrier and find out if the claim was received
   b. Rebill the insurance company
   c. Check on the processing status of the claim with the carrier
   d. Send an overdue notice
   e. Both a and c
5. When is the most appropriate time to discuss fees and the patient's financial concerns?
   a. When services are rendered
   b. When scheduling an appointment
   c. By mail after services are rendered
   d. When the insurance company does not pay the fee
6. The Truth-in-Lending Act is also known as what?
   a. Consumer Protection Act of 1967
   b. Fair Debt Collection Practice Act
   c. Patient Bankruptcy Protection Act
   d. Accurate Billing and Collection Act
   e. Fair Financial Treatment Act
7. The charge slip is also known by what other name?
   a. Ledger
   b. Encounter form
   c. Day sheet
   d. CMS-1500
8. What step should be taken when a patient files for bankruptcy?
   a. There is little likelihood that the debt can be collected
   b. It is best to close the account and identify the loss
   c. File a proof-of-claim form and provide a copy of the patient's outstanding account to the bankruptcy court
   d. Take the account to small claims court
   e. File a claim with the Consumer Protection Agency
9. What should you consider in determining how aggressive to be in debt collections?
   a. The previous month's billing backlog
   b. Production efficiency
   c. The terms of the insured's policy
   d. The value of the debt owed
10. Chapter 13 bankruptcy is otherwise known as what?
    a. Wage-earner's bankruptcy
    b. Farmer's bankruptcy
    c. Fair Lending bankruptcy
    d. Allowable debt bankruptcy
    e. Reorganization of debtor bankruptcy

LEARNING APPLICATION

Critical Thinking

1. An elderly widow covered only by Medicare Parts A and B is a patient in your clinic. You know her resources are limited. She receives a very small pension and Social Security benefits. She is facing hip replacement that will involve surgery, hospital care, rehabilitation care prior to her return to her apartment, and outpatient physical therapy. Describe what steps your clinic might take to ease her financial burden for this much needed care.

2. You are making a collections call. You follow all the rules and you are gracious in your approach. Before you realize what is happening, however, you have listened to a tale of woe, the patient is in tears, and you want to write your own check for the balance due. What happened? What will you do now?

3. Collections are an activity that many medical assistants shy away from and prefer not to do. What factors contribute to that feeling?

4. When the clinic manager calls a patient regarding a past-due account, she is told by the patient, "I'm not about to pay that bill. The treatment made my pain worse, not better." What steps might be taken now?

Hands-on Activity

Complete the charge slip for Charles Williams's clinic visit, based on the information below.

Charles Williams, 62 years old, is a new patient of Dr. Winston Lewis at Inner City Health Care. On July 1, 20XX, just 5 days before the patient's birthday, Charles comes to see Dr. Lewis for an appointment with a chief complaint of intermittent, irregular heartbeats (palpitations), dizziness, and chest pain. Dr. Lewis performs a comprehensive physical examination and orders several tests, including an ECG, complete blood count (CBC), and urinalysis with microscopy. The total fee for the clinic visit and tests is $345—$200 for the physical examination, $75 for the ECG, $25 for the urinalysis, $25 for venipuncture, and $20 for the CBC—which Charles pays for by check at the time of service. Charles is insured by a private carrier, All-American Insurance Company, group #333210, ID number 112-45-9980, which he receives through his employer, High Tech Computer Group. Dr. Lewis asks Ellen Armstrong, CMA (AAMA), to schedule a return appointment in exactly a week to go over the results of Charles's tests. Ellen schedules the appointment and prepares a charge slip for Charles's visit. She refers to his patient information sheet for the correct personal information. Charles Williams lives at 123 Greenside Street, Northborough, OH 12346.

DATE	PATIENT	SERVICE CODE	FEES CHARGE	CREDITS PAID	CREDITS ADJ.	BALANCE DUE	PREVIOUS BALANCE	NAME	RECEIPT NO.

THIS IS YOUR RECEIPT ____________
AND/OR A STATEMENT OF YOUR ACCOUNT TO DATE ____________

OFFICE VISITS AND PROCEDURES								
99211	EST PT - MINIMAL OV	1			HOSPITAL VISIT	14		
99212	EST PT - BRIEF OV	2			EMERGENCY	15		
99213	EST PT - INTERMEDIATE OV	3			CONSULTATION	16		
99214	EST PT - EXTENDED OV	4		93000	EKG	17		
99215	EST PT - COMPREHENSIVE OV	5		93224	ELECTROCARDIOGRAPHIC MONITORING	18		
99201	NEW PT - BRIEF OV	6		93307	ECHOCARDIOGRAPHY	19		
99202	NEW PT - INTERMEDIATE OV	7		85025	CBC	20		
99203	NEW PT - EXTENDED OV	8		81000	URINALYSIS WITH MICROSCOPY	21		
99204	NEW PT - COMPLEX OV	9		36415	ROUTINE VENIPUNCTURE	22		
99205	NEW PT - COMPREHENSIVE OF	10		71020	RADIOLOGY EXAM-CHEST-2 VIEWS	23		
99238	HOSPITAL DISCHARGE	11		30300	REMOVE FOR. BODY-INTRANASAL	24		
99025	NEW PT - SURGERY PROC. PRIMARY	12				25		
	NURSING HOME VISIT	13				26		

AUTHORIZATION TO RELEASE INFORMATION: I HEREBY AUTHORIZE THE UNDERSIGNED PHYSICIAN TO RELEASE ANY INFORMATION ACQUIRED IN THE COURSE OF MY EXAMINATION OR TREATMENT.
SIGNED (PATIENT, OR PARENT IF MINOR)

____________ DATE ____________

PLACE OF SERVICE ☒ OFFICE ☐ OTHER ____________

DIAGNOSIS OR SYMPTOMS ____________

DOCTOR'S SIGNATURE ____________

PATIENT'S NAME ____________ ☒ M ☐ F

ADDRESS

CITY STATE ZIP

RELATIONSHIP BIRTHDATE

SUBSCRIBER OR POLICY HOLDER

☐ MEDICARE ☐ MEDICAID ☐ BLUE SHIELD ☐ 65-SP.

INSURANCE CARRIER

AGREEMENT #

GROUP #

D - OTHER SERVICES

NEXT APPOINTMENT ____________ AT ____________ AM (PM)

RETURN ______ DAYS ______ (WEEKS) ______ MONTHS

Inner City Health Care
8600 Main St, SK 201
River City, NY 01234
(123) 555-0326

03626

Role-Play Activity

In pairs, role play a collection call using the information in Figure 19-5 in your text. One student should role play the medical assistant, and one should be Patient O'Keefe. At the conclusion of the role-play, the "medical assistant" and "patient" should each discuss how it felt to be the person in that role. Then have the students switch roles and perform the scenario again, with the same type of discussion afterward.

ATTRIBUTES OF PROFESSIONALISM

Some patients feel that medicine and money should never mix; however, a medical clinic is a business and must conduct itself as such. This means that collecting the copayment prior to the visit makes the most business sense. This means that collecting on amounts due from patients after their insurance has paid keeps the clinic financially viable.

In your journal write down phrases you might use in a variety of collections activities (for example, collecting a co-payment, contacting a patient about a check returned NSF, setting up a payment schedule for a noncovered service). It might help to put yourself in the patient's situation and think about a time or times when you paid a bill late or did not pay it until the following month. What was your reason(s)? How were you contacted/treated by the party to whom you owed the payment? Does this change your initial reaction and steps you would take? Consider how your provider will view your ability to keep current on accounts receivables.

Name ______________________ Date ________ Score ________

CHAPTER **20**

Accounting Practices

VOCABULARY BUILDER

Misspelled Words

Find the words below that are misspelled; circle them, and correctly spell them in the spaces provided. Then match the vocabulary words to the appropriate definitions below.

accounting	cash bases	income statement
accounts payible	check register	libility
accounts recievable ratio	collection ratio	owner's equity
accrual basis	cost analisys	trial balance
assets	cost ratio	utilazation review
balance sheet	fixed costs	varieble cost

__________________ __________________ __________________

__________________ __________________ __________________

__________________ __________________ __________________

1. ______________ Financial statement showing net profit or loss
2. ______________ Cost that varies in direct proportion to patient volume
3. ______________ Categorizes and records all checks written
4. ______________ Formula that measures the speed in which outstanding accounts are paid
5. ______________ The purpose of this is to determine the cost of each service
6. ______________ An itemized statement of assets, liabilities, and owner's equity; also called the statement of financial condition
7. ______________ System of reporting income where income is recognized at the time the money is collected
8. ______________ Cost that does not vary in total as the number of patients varies

9. ______________________ System of monitoring the financial status of a facility and the financial results of its activities, providing information for decision making

10. ______________________ Debt and other financial obligations for which one is responsible

11. ______________________ Formula that shows the percentage of outstanding debt collected

12. ______________________ Properties of value that are owned by a business entity

13. ______________________ Created by totaling debit balances and credit balances to make sure that total debits equal total credits

14. ______________________ The amount by which a business's assets exceed the business's liabilities

15. ______________________ Formula that shows the cost of a procedure or service and helps determine the financial value of maintaining certain services

16. ______________________ System of reporting income where income is reported at the time charges are generated

17. ______________________ A review of medical services before they can be performed

LEARNING REVIEW

Short Answer

1. There are a variety of methods used for financial management in the clinic. Name three of the bookkeeping systems that are appropriate for use in a medical clinic.

____

____

2. Medical software packages can code information obtained in the clinic for use in a database. When completing insurance claim forms or generating reports, the software has the capability to include the most common procedural and diagnostic codes. What other kinds of codes can a computerized accounting system generate that will facilitate the billing?

____

____

3. Practice management software can also be used in the preparation of financial documents. Name four financial documents.

____

4. Name three ways computer service bureaus handle accounts from medical facilities.

____

____

____

____

5. Identify at least four steps to take to reduce the chance of embezzlement.

____

____

____

____

6. To protect the practice from financial loss, providers can purchase fidelity bonds. Name and describe the three kinds of bonds. Place an *X* in front of the one that offers the most assurance.

1.	
2.	
3.	

7. How might the clinic manager use expense data from the income statement?

____

____

8. Why is it important to implement and track budgets for specific categories of income and expenses in the ambulatory care setting?

____

____

Matching I

Match the appropriate noncomputerized bookkeeping system to the following duties performed by the medical assistant.

A. Single-entry

B. Pegboard

C. Double-entry

_____ 1. Clinic manager Walter Seals, CMA (AAMA), was responsible for implementing a computer system at Inner City Urgent Care. Before the computerized accounting program was put into effect, the urgent care center relied on a manual system of checks and balances that allowed the provider-employers to keep a firm hold on the relationship between the facility's assets and the sum of liabilities and net worth.

_____ 2. During a temporary week-long down period in the computer system at Inner City Health Care while a system upgrade is being installed, administrative medical assistant Ellen Armstrong, CMAS (AMT), completes each day's financial transactions in a daily journal, then transfers this information to the ledger through the posting process. The information will be entered into the computer once the system is up and running again.

_____ 3. When the patient returns the charge slip to the reception desk after an examination, administrative medical assistant Ellen Armstrong carefully replaces and lines up the charge slip with the patient's name on the day sheet, then correctly inserts the ledger card under the last page of the charge slip. She proceeds to enter the total charges due and any patient payments.

Fixed and Variable Costs Exercise

Fixed costs are expenses that do not vary in total as the number of patients seen by the medical practice grows or shrinks. Variable costs are expenses that are directly affected by patient volume. From the list below, identify expenses that qualify as fixed costs (FC) and those that are variable costs (VC).

_____ 1. Interpreting laboratory test results

_____ 2. Annual depreciation of the cost of an automatic electrocardiograph (ECG) machine

_____ 3. Medical benefits for the clinic staff

_____ 4. Purchase of reagent test strips for urinalysis

_____ 5. Magazine subscriptions for the facility reception area

_____ 6. Monthly telephone expenses

_____ 7. Medical journal subscriptions for the providers

_____ 8. Purchase of a HemoCue blood glucose system

_____ 9. Weekly printing cost of a patient education brochure

_____ 10. Purchase of open-shelf lateral files

_____ 11. Adding a new position, such as a clinical medical assistant, to the clinic staff

_____ 12. Property taxes on the medical facility building and grounds

_____ 13. The monthly cost of janitorial services

_____ 14. Purchase of disposable needle–syringe units

_____ 15. Disposable paper gowns for patient examinations

CERTIFICATION REVIEW

These questions are designed to mimic the certification examination. Select the best response.

1. What is the system that is based on the accounting principle that assets equal liabilities plus owner's equity?
   a. Single-entry system
   b. Double-entry system
   c. Standard of billing services bureaus
   d. Accounts receivable accounting principles

2. Of the following statements, which is false?
   a. Double-entry bookkeeping is expensive
   b. Double-entry bookkeeping is accurate
   c. Double-entry bookkeeping is more time consuming than other methods
   d. Double-entry bookkeeping has checks and balances in place
   e. Double-entry bookkeeping has built-in accuracy controls

3. Which of the following is owner's equity *not* the same as?
   a. Net worth
   b. Proprietorship
   c. Capital
   d. Accounts payable

4. Bonds may be purchased to protect the practice from which of the following?
   a. Embezzlement
   b. Financial loss
   c. Malpractice suits
   d. Stock market loss
   e. Both a and b

5. Which of the following is a capability of a practice management system?
   a. Process insurance claims electronically
   b. Manage payroll and purchases
   c. Generate financial records
   d. All of the above

6. Examples of variable costs include all of the following *except* what?
   a. Clinical supplies
   b. Equipment costs
   c. Depreciation
   d. Laboratory procedures
   e. Payroll and benefits

7. How is the trial balance created?
   a. Collecting data from the current year and previous year and converting them into a ratio
   b. Totaling debit balances and credit balances to confirm that total debits equal total credits
   c. Reporting outside revenue sources and overhead expenses
   d. Recording two sets of entries, such as increase in assets and increase in liabilities

8. Why should providers purchase fidelity bonds?
   a. They are worth the price.
   b. They provide a sense of security.
   c. They lessen the chances of embezzlement.
   d. They will reimburse the practice for any monetary loss caused by the practice's employees.
   e. All of the above

9. Which of the following is a reason a proper contract should be negotiated and signed with any computer and billing service bureau?
   a. It is considered a legal document.
   b. It ensures confidentiality and strict privacy of patient information.
   c. It is required for HIPAA compliance.
   d. Both b and c

10. A hospital cost report for Medicare is considered a part of which of the following?
    a. Financial accounting
    b. Managerial accounting
    c. Cost accounting
    d. Cost analysis
    e. Cost ratio

LEARNING APPLICATION

Critical Thinking

1. Discuss the pros and cons of on-site computerized accounting software or a practice management system and a computer service bureau.

2. The accounting equation can be reported in more than one formula. It can be stated as:
   a. assets = liabilities + owner's equity, or
   b. assets − liabilities = owner's equity

   Is one easier to interpret? Why or why not? Add some totals of your choice to illustrate.

3. Recall from previous chapters and other studies in which you may be involved some basic guidelines for using computers/software programs in the clinic. Identify these. What is one critical procedure that is done quite regularly, especially at the end of a project or the end of the day?

Case Studies

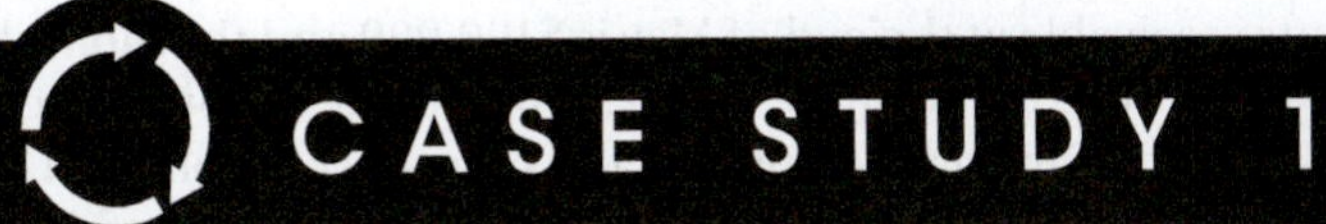

CASE STUDY 1

When Inner City Health Care agreed to accept individuals covered by a large managed care organization, the decision of the provider-owners was based on a complete financial analysis and projection of the expected effects the new patient load would have on the medical practice. As a result, the group practice added a second clinic manager and a new clinical medical assistant to the existing staff.

CASE STUDY REVIEW QUESTIONS

1. As Inner City Health Care absorbs the new managed care patients into the practice, what can the provider-owners do to determine whether their financial analysis and projection were accurate?

2. Once the practice has assembled financial data on the effects of the new patient load, how will these data be used?

3. What beneficial effects might the addition of a clinical medical assistant have on the clinic?

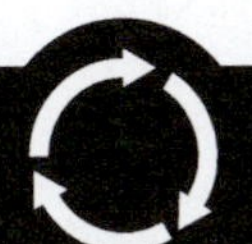

CASE STUDY 2

A group practice of radiologists charges $225 for a routine mammogram. Total expenses related to the mammogram procedure equal $30,000 per month, and the practice performs a monthly average of 200 mammograms.

CASE STUDY REVIEW QUESTIONS

1. What is the average cost ratio for the mammogram procedure? (Show your calculations in the space provided).

2. Given the cost to patients for mammograms, is the group practice making a profit or loss on performing mammograms? What amount is the profit or loss per mammogram? What amount is the profit or loss for the entire month?

Hands-on Activities

1. At Inner City Health Care, the total accounts receivable at the end of May is $100,000 and the monthly receipts total is $75,000; the total accounts receivable at the end of June is $82,000 and the monthly receipts total is $31,000; the total accounts receivable at the end of July is $86,000 and the monthly receipts total is $20,000; the total accounts receivable at the end of August is $93,000 and the monthly receipts total is $45,000. What is the accounts receivable ratio for each month? Show your calculations in the space provided. Which month has the healthiest accounts receivable ratio? Why?

May: ___	July: ___
June: ____	August: ___

2. For the month of September, receipts at Inner City Health Care totaled $35,000. The Medicare/Medicaid adjustment for the month was $1,750, and the managed care adjustment was $4,500. Total charges for the month of September equaled $53,000. What is the collection ratio for the month of September? (Show your calculation in the space provided.)

3. For the month of October, receipts at Inner City Health Care totaled $41,000. The Medicare/Medicaid adjustment for the month was $2,000; the Workers' Compensation adjustment was $750; and the managed care adjustment was $4,700. Total charges for October equaled $55,000. What is the collection ratio for the month of October? (Show your calculation in the space provided.)

4. Income statements reveal the cumulative profit and total expenses for each month. Monthly income and expenses are then added to arrive at year-to-date totals, which are compared with the annual budget for particular income and expense categories. Use the following information to complete the expense analysis table for the first-quarter office expense costs of Inner City Health Care. The total office expense budget for the year is $20,000 divided evenly per quarter.

Telephone expenses	January $323.46
	February $425.93
	March $393.87
Postage and mail expenses	January $725.45
	February $550.90
	March $601.33
Office supply expenses	January $1,200.62
	February $325.45
	March $446.26
Yearly budget	Telephone expenses $4,000
	Postage and mail expenses $8,000
	Office supply expenses $8,000

Office Expenses	January	February	March	Year to Date	Budget for Year
Telephone	______	______	______	______	______
Postage	______	______	______	______	______
Office supplies	______	______	______	______	______
TOTALS	______	______	______	______	______

ATTRIBUTES OF PROFESSIONALISM

Previous chapters (16 through 19) have addressed the topics of proper daily bookkeeping, financial practices, accurate coding, processing of insurance forms, and the efficient management of collection on accounts. All of these functions are essential to obtaining maximum reimbursement and creating profitability for the clinic. This chapter ties many of these elements together and creates a total picture of their interdependence.

Reflecting on what you have learned throughout the finance-related chapters, do you feel as though you have a better understanding of how your duties as a medical assistant tie in? Does what you have learned give you a different perspective on how you handle your personal finances? In your journal write at least three Attributes of Professionalism that you feel are most related to the clinic's financial practices. Describe in detail your reasoning and cite examples.

____

____

____

____

____

____

Name ____________________ Date ________ Score ________

CHAPTER 21

Infection Control and Medical Asepsis

VOCABULARY BUILDER

Misspelled Words

Find the words below that are misspelled; circle them, and then correctly spell them in the space provided. Then insert the vocabulary terms into the sentences below. Each word will be used once.

aseptic	humoral immunity	palyative
bascili	immunoglobulins	parenteral
bloodborne pathigen	isolation	pruritis
communicable	malaise	resistence
coryza	microorganisms	sputim
epidemic	nosecomial	vector
____________	____________	____________
____________	____________	____________

1. Antibodies are called ____________.
2. ____________ is associated with circulating antibodies that fight infection.
3. An acute, contagious respiratory infection is called ____________ or rhinitis.
4. Infections that are acquired from the hands of health care professionals are known as ____________ infections.
5. ____________ is a medical term meaning freedom from any infectious material.
6. Diseases that are carried by animals or insects are spread by ____________ transmission.
7. Gram-negative ____________ cause infections including pneumonia, bloodstream infections, wound or surgical site infections, and meningitis in health care settings.

8. Viral infections are difficult to treat. Most of the care provided is designed to relieve symptoms and is known as ______________________ treatment.

9. When there is a sudden outbreak of disease or an ______________________, the CDC investigates the cause and methods of control.

10. The overuse or misuse of antibiotics has been linked to the emergence and spread of microorganisms which have developed ______________________ to them, rendering treatment ineffective and posing a serious risk to public health.

11. Diseases that are easily spread by contact with an infected person are known as ______________________ diseases.

12. ______________________ is the liquid that comes from your respiratory tract when you cough.

13. ______________________ represents one of several measures that can be taken to implement infection control.

14. Contact with blood should be avoided because ______________________ are common causes of disease processes.

15. Medications administered other than orally are considered ______________________ medications.

16. ______________________ is a feeling of weakness, overall discomfort, illness, or simply not feeling well.

17. ______________________ are microscopic living organisms that are capable of causing illness and disease.

18. ______________________ is severe itching of the skin.

LEARNING REVIEW

Short Answer

1. List two types of immune responses and describe the process of each.

____

____

____

____

2. Describe the handling of infectious waste.

____

____

____

____

3. What are the five stages of infectious disease? Describe each.

____

____

____

____

4. What are the four items that are considered personal protective equipment? Describe each one.

5. What factors influence the host's susceptibility?

Matching I

Identify the causative agent of each of the following diseases. Place a B beside those that are caused by bacteria and a V beside those that are caused by a viral agent.

_____ A. Lyme disease

_____ B. Avian flu

_____ C. AIDS

_____ D. Pertussis

_____ E. Rubella

_____ F. Chicken pox

_____ G. Toxic shock syndrome

_____ H. SARS

_____ I. VRE

_____ J. MRSA

Matching II

Match each of the following types of transmission with the correct definition.

Contact transmission

Droplet transmission

Airborne transmission

Vector transmission

Fomite transmission

Bloodborne transmission

________________ 1. Involves animals and insects that are capable of transmitting diseases

________________ 2. Microorganisms are transferred from an inanimate object such as a doorknob, table, or medical equipment

________________ 3. Occurs when respiratory droplets are generated by a patient who is coughing, sneezing, or talking

________________ 4. Occurs when microorganisms are suspended in the air for long periods of time

________________ 5. Physical contact between an infected person, or his or her body fluids, and a susceptible person that results in a transfer of microorganisms

________________ 6. Infected blood enters a susceptible host through exposure to blood or body fluids

CERTIFICATION REVIEW

These questions are designed to mimic the certification examination. Select the best response.

1. The use of biologic agents such as pathogenic microorganisms to do damage to a society is considered which of the following?
   a. Chain of infection
   b. Disinfection
   c. Bioterrorism
   d. Sterilization

2. Which of the following is a common way to accidentally come in contact with blood and body fluids?
   a. Phlebotomy
   b. Administering an injection
   c. Assisting with suturing or removal of sutures
   d. Performing wound irrigation
   e. All of the above

3. People, equipment, supplies, and food and water are considered which part of the chain of infection?
   a. Portal of entry
   b. Susceptible host
   c. Reservoir
   d. Portal of exit

4. A person that is capable of contracting a pathogenic organism is called which of the following?
   a. Means of transmission
   b. Portal of exit
   c. Reservoir
   d. Susceptible host
   e. Infectious agent

5. What is the body's first line of defense?
   a. Hand washing
   b. Intact skin
   c. Immune system
   d. Antibiotics

6. The most important aspect of infection control is which of the following?
   a. Immune response
   b. Sterilization
   c. Hand washing
   d. Mode of transmission
   e. Use of biohazard disposal units

7. The portal of exit is a part of the chain of infection. The best description of the portal of exit is which of the following?
   a. The method by which an infectious agent leaves the reservoir
   b. People, equipment, supplies, water, food, and animals or insects
   c. Microorganisms that are the causative agents of disease
   d. Specific ways in which microorganisms travel from one place to another

8. Which of the following is a barrier that protects our bodies from infection?
   a. Skin and mucous membranes
   b. Body excretions and secretions
   c. Immune system
   d. Leukocytes
   e. All of the above

9. There are steps that must be followed to allow the spread of infectious disease. What is this process called?
   a. Bacteria
   b. Chain of infection
   c. Infection control
   d. Disinfection

10. If an employee has suffered an occupational exposure, how long must that medical record be kept?
    a. The length of employment plus 10 years
    b. The length of employment plus 20 years
    c. The length of employment plus 30 years
    d. The length of employment only
    e. As long as the practice is open and seeing patients

LEARNING APPLICATION

Critical Thinking

1. Analyze the importance of infection control and give five examples of how a medical assistant would practice infection control in the ambulatory care setting.

2. Your patient has a draining wound. After you change the dressing, explain how to prevent the transmission of microorganisms from the wound and dressing to you or to another patient.

3. Give an example of how the proper disposal of contaminated objects can break a link in the chain of infection.

4. You notice a co-worker sanitizing surgical instruments in preparation for sterilization. He did not scrub the serrations on the instruments well. What will be the result of his improper sanitization technique? Explain your answer.

5. Describe eight procedures/techniques that you could perform or assist with on a patient that could expose you to bloodborne pathogens.

6. What alternative do you have if you do not have access to soap and water after performing a procedure on a patient?

7. Explain the differences between sanitation and disinfection.

8. Considering the growth requirements for pathogens, describe how to discourage bacterial growth in the patient examination room.

Case Studies

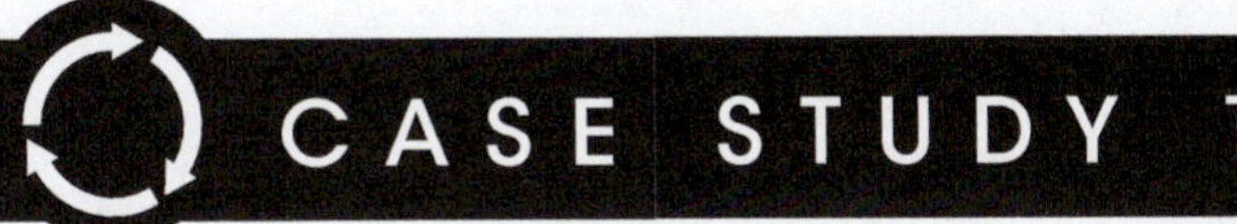

Your provider-employer asks you to help develop an exposure control plan. Include measures the employer must take to eliminate or lessen employees' risk for exposure to blood or other potentially infectious materials.

CASE STUDY REVIEW QUESTIONS

1. What should be included in an exposure control plan?

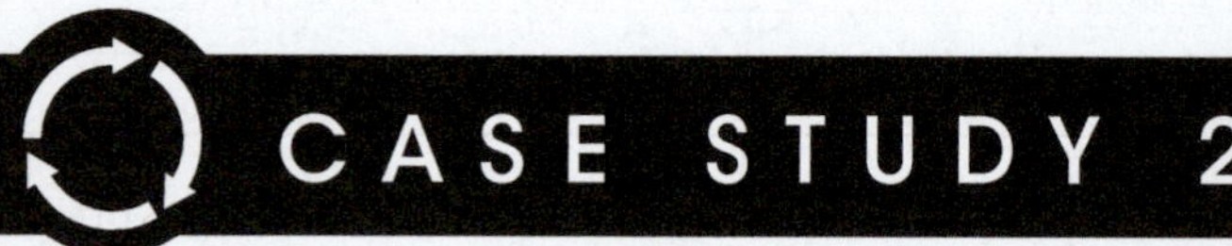

CASE STUDY 2

Veronica Hernandez, a medical assisting extern at Inner City Health Care, attends to patient procedures and examinations under the supervision of clinic manager Marilyn Johnson, CMA (AAMA). Although Veronica is careful to follow all infection control methods during patient care, severe dermatitis has developed on her hands. She is concerned that this condition, which has not responded to creams and lotions, is related to the latex gloves she wears during procedures.

CASE STUDY REVIEW QUESTIONS

1. Discuss the possible causes of Veronica's symptoms.

____

____

____

____

2. Suggest a course of action that both addresses Veronica's condition and maintains the proper degree of asepsis.

____

____

____

Hands-on Activities

Complete the following forms with the indicated information.

1. Place an *X* in the correct category of waste disposal for each item described.

Item	Regular Trash	Red Bag Trash	Sharps Container
Empty bottle of alcohol-based hand rub			
Soiled adult diaper with formed stool			
Used tongue depressor			
Empty IV bag			
Used syringe with needle attached			
Used sanitation wipe			
Used lancet			
Used blood glucose strip			
Soiled gown from dressing change			
Nonsterile gloves after dressing change			
Urine dipstick			
Used razor			
Cotton-tipped swab after wound cleaning			

Blood spill kit after use			
Disposable suction containers after use			
Gauze sponges after using to control bleeding			
Infant diaper			
Suture with needle attached			
Broken glass slide			
Facial tissue after use by patient with influenza			
Catheter and catheter bag after removal from patient			

2. You checked the emergency cleanup spill kits in all your exam rooms and in the clinical laboratory. You made sure they were complete, had not expired, were intact without tears, and were ready to use when needed. Make notation of your checks on the following form.

Location	Checked by	Date	Assessment Action taken
Exam Room #1			
Exam Room #2			
Exam Room #3			
Lab Station #1			
Lab Kit #2			

3. You are a clinical medical assistant at Inner City Health Care. You arrived at work this morning at 9:00 A.M. At 11:30 A.M., while assisting Dr. Amy Cox to suture a 3 cm laceration on the right forearm of a patient, you received an accidental posterior to anterior needle stick of your right index finger. The needle stick occurred while you were clearing the Mayo stand of the laceration repair instruments. Report the incident using the following form. (*NOTE:* For reporting purposes, identify fellow medical assistant Nancy McFarland as the person who completed the form.)

OSHA's Form 301
Injury and Illness Incident Report

Attention: This form contains information relating to employee health and must be used in a manner that protects the confidentiality of employees to the extent possible while the information is being used for occupational safety and health purposes.

U.S. Department of Labor
Occupational Safety and Health Administration

Form approved OMB no. 1218-0176

This *Injury and Illness Incident Report* is one of the first forms you must fill out when a recordable work-related injury or illness has occurred. Together with the *Log of Work-Related Injuries and Illnesses* and the accompanying *Summary*, these forms help the employer and OSHA develop a picture of the extent and severity of work-related incidents.

Within 7 calendar days after you receive information that a recordable work-related injury or illness has occurred, you must fill out this form or an equivalent. Some state workers' compensation, insurance, or other reports may be acceptable substitutes. To be considered an equivalent form, any substitute must contain all the information asked for on this form.

According to Public Law 91-596 and 29 CFR 1904, OSHA's recordkeeping rule, you must keep this form on file for 5 years following the year to which it pertains.

If you need additional copies of this form, you may photocopy and use as many as you need.

Completed by ______________________

Title ______________________

Phone (____)______-________ Date ____/____/____

Information about the employee

1) Full name ______________________

2) Street ______________________

City ______________ State ______ ZIP ______

3) Date of birth ____/____/____

4) Date hired ____/____/____

5) ☐ Male
☐ Female

Information about the physician or other health care professional

6) Name of physician or other health care professional ______________________

7) If treatment was given away from the worksite, where was it given?

Facility ______________________

Street ______________________

City ______________ State ______ ZIP ______

8) Was employee treated in an emergency room?
☐ Yes
☐ No

9) Was employee hospitalized overnight as an in-patient?
☐ Yes
☐ No

Information about the case

10) Case number from the *Log* ____________ *(Transfer the case number from the Log after you record the case.)*

11) Date of injury or illness ____/____/____

12) Time employee began work ____________ AM / PM

13) Time of event ____________ AM / PM ☐ Check if time cannot be determined

14) ***What was the employee doing just before the incident occurred?*** Describe the activity, as well as the tools, equipment, or material the employee was using. Be specific. *Examples:* "climbing a ladder while carrying roofing materials"; "spraying chlorine from hand sprayer"; "daily computer key-entry."

15) ***What happened?*** Tell us how the injury occurred. *Examples:* "When ladder slipped on wet floor, worker fell 20 feet"; "Worker was sprayed with chlorine when gasket broke during replacement"; "Worker developed soreness in wrist over time."

16) ***What was the injury or illness?*** Tell us the part of the body that was affected and how it was affected; be more specific than "hurt," "pain," or sore." *Examples:* "strained back"; "chemical burn, hand"; "carpal tunnel syndrome."

17) ***What object or substance directly harmed the employee?*** *Examples:* "concrete floor"; "chlorine"; "radial arm saw." *If this question does not apply to the incident, leave it blank.*

18) ***If the employee died, when did death occur?*** Date of death ____/____/____

Public reporting burden for this collection of information is estimated to average 22 minutes per response, including time for reviewing instructions, searching existing data sources, gathering and maintaining the data needed, and completing and reviewing the collection of information. Persons are not required to respond to the collection of information unless it displays a current valid OMB control number. If you have any comments about this estimate or any other aspects of this data collection, including suggestions for reducing this burden, contact: US Department of Labor, OSHA Office of Statistical Analysis, Room N-3644, 200 Constitution Avenue, NW, Washington, DC 20210. Do not send the completed forms to this office.

ATTRIBUTES OF PROFESSIONALISM

In the course of caring for patients as a medical assistant, it is likely that you will be exposed to patients who have life-threatening infectious diseases. What Attributes of Professionalism might you utilize to protect your health and maintain a respectful manner when providing care? Evaluate your belief systems and record methods of demonstrating empathy in this situation.

Name ______________________ Date __________ Score __________

CHAPTER 24

The Physical Examination

VOCABULARY REVIEW

Misspelled Words

Find the words below that are misspelled; circle them, and then correctly spell them in the space provided. Then identify the vocabulary term most appropriate for each example below from a patient's physical examination.

ataxia	labirynthitis	symmetry
bruits	paller	tinnitus
cianosis	piorrhea	vertigo
jaundice	schleroderma	vertiligo

______________________ ______________________ ______________________

______________________ ______________________ ______________________

1. During a physical examination of Louise Kipperley, a 48-year-old woman, Dr. Esposito notices that Louise's facial skin has become tight and atrophied, suggesting possible ________________.
2. Leo McKay comes to Inner City Health Care with mouth pain. Dr. Reynolds examines Leo's mouth and discovers ________________, which is discharge of pus from the gums around the teeth.
3. Medical assistant Liz Corbin, CMA (AAMA), observes the gait of Geraldine Potter, a 36-year-old woman diagnosed with multiple sclerosis. Geraldine's gait is lurching and unsteady, with her feet widely placed. Liz charts this as ________________.
4. Annette Samuels is diagnosed with hepatitis B virus (HBV) by Dr. Lewis. Among Annette's symptoms, noted by Dr. Lewis during the physical examination, was ________________, a distinct yellowing of Annette's skin and the whites of her eyes.
5. Lenny Taylor, an older adult male with Alzheimer disease, is brought to Inner City Health Care by his son George. Apparently, Lenny has had problems breathing. Dr. King observes ________________, a bluish color in Lenny's skin.

6. After performing a routine venipuncture procedure on patient Rhonda Campbell, Sam Huckaby, CMA (AAMA), notices that all color has drained from Rhonda's face. He assumes that her ________________ is due to a psychological reaction to the venipuncture, so he has her lie down on the examination table for a few minutes until her color improves.

7. Abigail Johnson's 28-year-old granddaughter Lucy comes in for an examination with Dr. King after observing white patches of depigmentation, or ________________, on her hand. "Is this what Michael Jackson had?" she asks Dr. King.

8. While performing a complete physical examination on patient Ann Cook, Dr. King listens for abnormal sounds, or ________________, from vital organs while auscultating her abdomen.

9. During a routine physical examination of Joanna Rowe, a young woman who is confined to a wheelchair, Dr. Lewis checks for balance—or ________________ of size, shape, and position—of body parts on opposite sides of her body.

10. Addi Mountjoy comes in to see Dr. King for ringing in her ears. Dr. King asks her if she is taking large doses of aspirin, which can cause ________________.

11. Ashley White's 6-year-old daughter, Brittney, who has been diagnosed with a case of the mumps, returns with her mother for a reexamination with Dr. Lewis when the child experiences a sensation that the room is spinning, caused by inflammation of the labyrinth, called ________________.

12. While her blood was being taken, Susan O'Donnell described the room as spinning, and she felt light-headed. ________________ is a common reaction to a stress-induced drop in blood pressure.

LEARNING REVIEW

Matching

Match the terms listed in Column A with the corresponding descriptions in Column B.

Column A	Column B
_____ 1. Auscultation	A. On his physical examination of Charles Williams, Dr. Winston Lewis looks at the patient to assess his general health, posture, body movements, skin, mannerisms, and care in grooming while verbally reviewing Charles's medical history with him.
_____ 2. Observation or inspection	B. Dr. Angie Esposito uses a stethoscope to listen to the bowel sounds that accompany peristalsis.
_____ 3. Manipulation	C. Dr. King performs range of motion exercises on patient Margaret Thomas, who is suspected of having Parkinson disease.
_____ 4. Mensuration	D. Dr. Rice taps Edith Leonard's chest to feel and hear the hollow quality expected from clear lungs.
_____ 5. Percussion	E. During Marissa O'Keefe's well-baby visit, chest and head circumference measurements are recorded in the patient's medical record.

Short Answer

1. Identify each entry below as a piece of medical equipment (ME), a laboratory procedure (LP), a body part (BP), or a patient illness or condition (PI). Then identify the correct component or sequence of the physical examination to which the entry relates. The first two entries have been completed for you as an example.

A. Sphygmomanometer	ME	Vital signs
B. Aphonia	PI	Speech
C. Lymph nodes	_____	________________
D. Edema	_____	________________
E. Anal fissures	_____	________________
F. Emphysema	_____	________________
G. Pharyngeal mirrors	_____	________________
H. Scrotum	_____	________________
I. Areola	_____	________________
J. Electrocardiography	_____	________________
K. Kyphosis	_____	________________
L. Dysphasia	_____	________________
M. Urinalysis	_____	________________
N. Achilles tendon	_____	________________
O. Tympanic membrane	_____	________________

2. Symmetry would be noted by using what method of assessment?

____

3. What is another term for the supine position, or the position assumed when lying face up?

____

4. *(Circle the correct answer)* Orthostatic hypotension occurs as blood pressure decreases/increases/normalizes.

5. What is the preferred position for administration of an enema or rectal suppository?

____

6. Determining the amount of flexion and extension of a patient's extremities would be which form of assessment?

____

Image Identification

Identify each of the positions shown in the photos below.

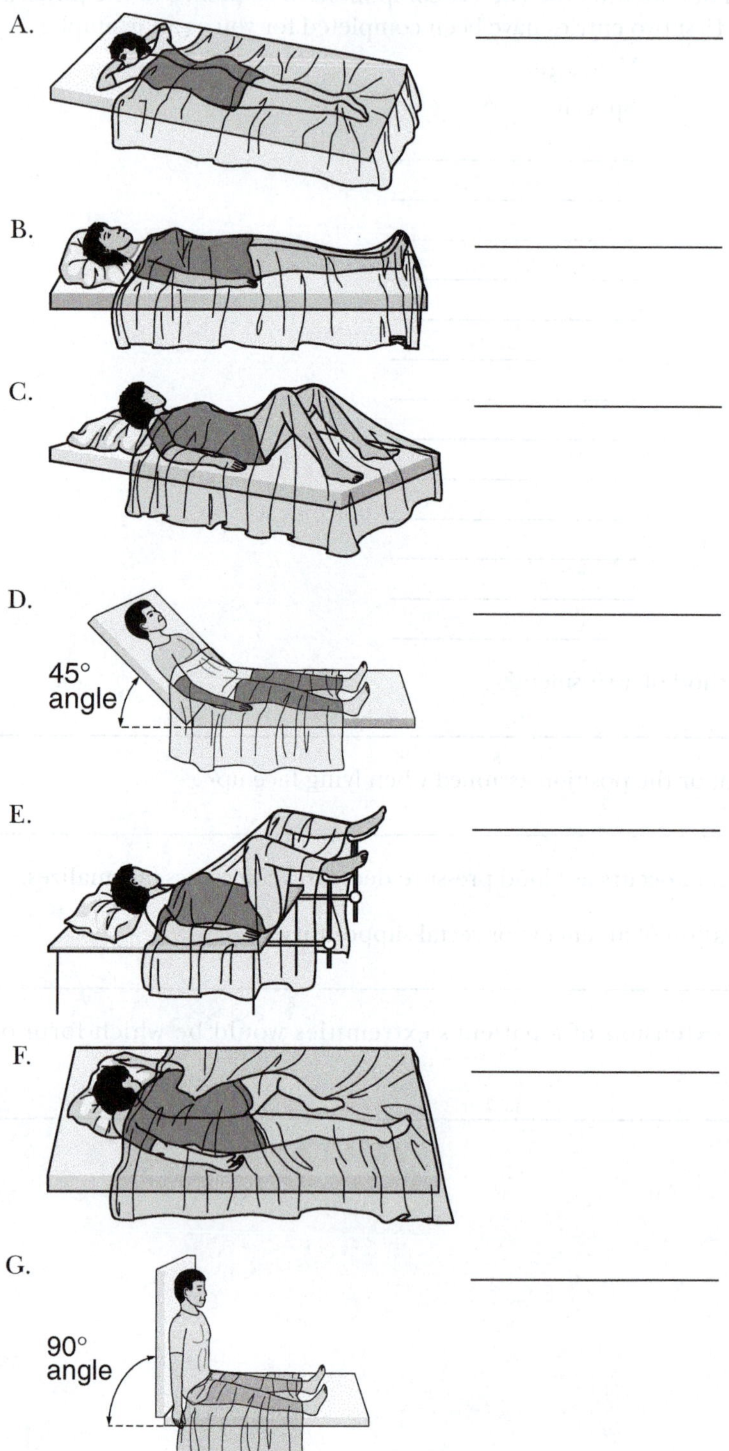

A. ____________________

B. ____________________

C. ____________________

D. ____________________

E. ____________________

F. ____________________

G. ____________________

CERTIFICATION REVIEW

These questions are designed to mimic the certification examination. Select the best response.

1. A patient having an examination of the abdomen should be placed in which position?
   a. Supine
   b. Prone
   c. Lithotomy
   d. Sims'

2. Listening to the patient's chest as he or she breathes is called which of the following?
   a. Auscultation
   b. Percussion
   c. Inspection
   d. Palpation
   e. Mensuration

3. Cyanosis is an indicator of diseases of which system?
   a. Gastrointestinal
   b. Respiratory
   c. Cardiovascular
   d. Both b and c

4. Which of the following is *not* a word used to describe skin color?
   a. Jaundice
   b. Cyanosis
   c. Bruits
   d. Pallor
   e. Flushing

5. Examination of the ears is an important aspect of a physical exam. Which of the following is *not* utilized when examining the ears?
   a. Ophthalmoscope
   b. Tuning fork
   c. Otoscope
   d. Audiometer

6. Which examination technique consists of eliciting sounds from the body by tapping?
   a. Observation
   b. Inspection
   c. Percussion
   d. Palpation
   e. Mensuration

7. The most comfortable position for patients with back or abdominal problems when lying on an exam table is what?
   a. Semi-Fowler's
   b. Supine
   c. Lithotomy
   d. Dorsal recumbent

8. Which examination includes internal genitalia, external genitalia, and rectal exam?
   a. Female genital
   b. Male genital
   c. Perinatal
   d. Both a and b
   e. None of the above

9. Which of the following are instructions that might be given to a patient during a breast exam?
   a. Place your hand behind your head.
   b. Take a deep breath.
   c. Please swallow.
   d. Close your right eye.

10. Auscultation, palpation, and mensuration are utilized to examine what area of the body?
    a. Abdomen
    b. Breast
    c. Heart
    d. Chest
    e. Extremities

LEARNING APPLICATION

Critical Thinking

1. Discuss the responsibilities of the medical assistant when preparing a patient for a physical examination.

____

____

____

____

____

____

2. Review the six methods used in the physical examination.

____

____

____

____

3. Explain the sequence of a physical examination.

____

(1) ____

____

(2) ____

____

4. Describe the cleaning process that the following instruments will need after their use in an examination:

   a. ______________________________

   ____

   b. ______________________________

   c. ______________________________

   d. ______________________________

   ____

5. List and describe the three sources of information the provider uses to aid in making a diagnosis.

   (1) ______________________________

   ____

   (2) ______________________________

   (3) ______________________________

   ____

6. List two procedures or tests the medical assistant might perform as part of the patient's physical examination.

   ____

   ____

   ____

Case Studies

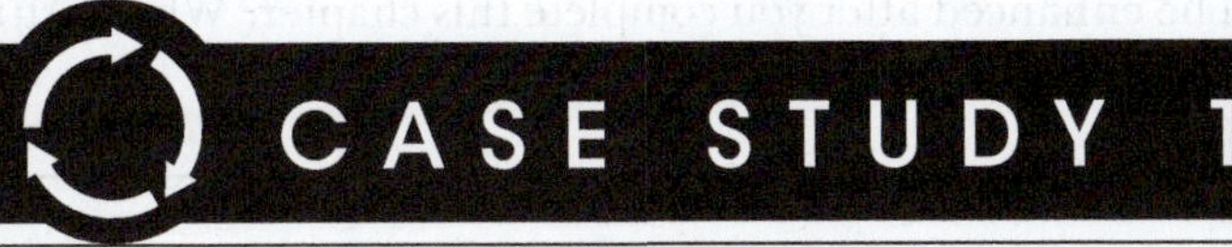

Holly Carmona brings her young daughter, Wren, to Heartland Pediatrics with a suspected case of mumps, which Wren's older sister is just recovering from. As Sarah Thomas, CMA (AAMA), helps the child remove her shirt for the examination, Wren becomes increasingly fearful and begins to cry. It is obvious the child is feverish and not feeling well.

CASE STUDY REVIEW QUESTIONS

1. What aspects of the physical exam will be important to make a diagnosis of mumps?

   ____

   ____

   ____

   ____

   ____

2. How can Sarah be the most helpful to the provider to allow ease of examination?

   ____

   ____

   ____

   ____

   ____

Role-Play Exercise

Using the list of patient positions from the textbook, practice placing your classmates into the various positions for examination. Pay special attention to knee and back problems and any physical limitations patients may have.

ATTRIBUTES OF PROFESSIONALISM

Think about the last time you went to see your primary care provider. As you answer the following questions and remember your personal experience(s), think about how your experience(s) will affect the way you treat your patients in the future. If you have no such personal experiences, try to imagine how you would feel and react.

1. Did you have to undress at all? How did that feel? Did you get cold or feel a bit awkward?

   ____

   ____

   ____

2. When you had your blood pressure taken, did the cuff cause pain or discomfort as it got tighter? Did you say something to the medical assistant or other staff? Do you think most patients speak up when they are uncomfortable?

   ____

   ____

   ____

3. Have you ever noticed a sick patient in a public place? What were the clues that told you the patient was sick? Do you think your skills of observation will be enhanced after you complete this chapter? Which Attributes of Professionalism will be most important to enhancing your skills of observation?

   ____

   ____

   ____

   ____

   ____

   ____

   ____

   ____

Name ________________________________ Date ________ Score ________

CHAPTER 25

Obstetrics and Gynecology

VOCABULARY REVIEW

Misspelled Words

Find the words below that are misspelled; circle them, and then correctly spell them in the space provided. Then fill in the blanks in the following sentences with the correct vocabulary terms from the list.

abortion	effacement	multigravida
amniotomy	ektopic	nullypara
Bartholyn glands	guestation	parturtion
colposcopy	hipoxia	pelvic inflammatory disease
coupling agent	hyperemesis gravidarum	placenta previa
cryosurgery	hysterosalpingogram	sickle cell anemia
delation	lokia	Tay–Sachs
dismenorrhea	meconium	trichomoniasis
dyspareunia		

________________ ________________ ________________

________________ ________________ ________________

________________ ________________ ________________

1. The provider instructs you to prepare the room for a ________________ in order to examine the patient's vagina and cervix using a lighted instrument that has magnification capabilities.

2. The diagnosis of ________________ results when the *Trichomonas* parasite is identified.

3. In order to enhance the penetration of sound waves through the tissue, especially when listening to the fetal heartbeat, a ________________ is applied to the mother's abdomen.

4. Ms. Eubanks is pregnant for the first time. For this reason, ________________ is recorded in her medical record to reflect this fact.

5. An ________________ may be performed if fetal membranes do not spontaneously rupture.

6. The first stool of the newborn, ______________________, may indicate fetal distress.

7. Ms. Ann Boyles is seen in the clinic today and reports that intercourse is painful. The medical term for this condition is ____________________.

8. Pregnant women with ______________________ vomit excessively and may become dehydrated and fail to gain weight appropriately.

9. Abnormal cells found on the cervix are commonly treated with a freezing technique known as ______________________.

LEARNING REVIEW

Short Answer

1. What branch of medicine treats the mother and fetus through all stages of labor, delivery, and postpartum?

____

2. List at least two signs/symptoms of preeclampsia.

____

____

____

3. Describe the dilation and curettage procedure and the indications for this procedure.

____

____

____

4. List some of the benefits of breast-feeding for the mother and the baby.

____

____

____

5. List and describe the six types of abortion.

____

____

____

____

____

6. Describe the emergency condition of placenta previa.

____

____

____

7. Describe Rh incompatibility and treatment options.

____

____

____

____

8. List and describe the three stages of labor.

____

____

____

9. Recall the screenings that are a usual part of an annual gynecologic exam.

____

Matching

Match each term in Column I to its description in Column II.

Column I	Column II
_____ 1. PID	A. Technique consisting of breathing exercises to ease and facilitate labor and delivery
_____ 2. Menopause	B. Painful menstruation
_____ 3. Endometriosis	C. The period from the end of the third stage of labor until involution of the uterus is complete
_____ 4. Ovarian cancer	D. Inflammatory disease of the pelvis involving some or all of the reproductive organs
_____ 5. Ovarian cysts	E. Sudden separation of the placenta from the uterine wall
_____ 6. Dysmenorrhea	F. Cysts located on the ovaries
_____ 7. Lamaze	G. A pituitary hormone that stimulates the muscles of the uterus to contract
_____ 8. Puerperium	H. Painful condition characterized by endometrial cells adhering to tissues and organs outside of the uterus
_____ 9. Placenta abruptio	I. Malignant cells found in the ovaries
_____ 10. Oxytocin	J. The end of menstruation

Image Labeling

Identify each part of the female reproductive system below. Describe each part and its function in the spaces provided. Use your medical dictionary if needed.

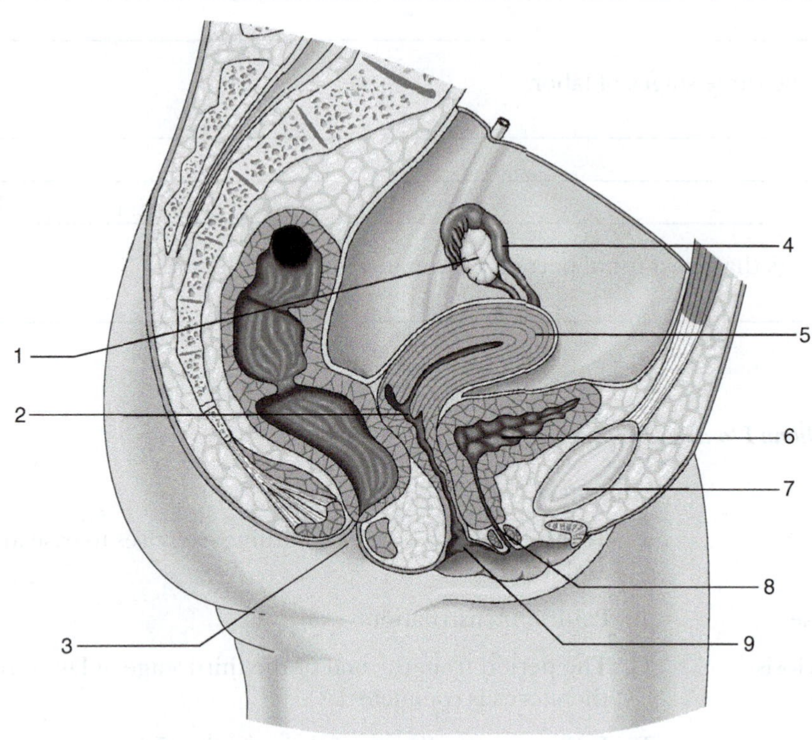

Part | **Description and Function**

1. ____________ ______________________________
2. ____________ ______________________________
3. ____________ ______________________________
4. ____________ ______________________________
5. ____________ ______________________________
6. ____________ ______________________________
7. ____________ ______________________________
8. ____________ ______________________________
9. ____________ ______________________________

CERTIFICATION REVIEW

These questions are designed to mimic the certification examination. Select the best response.

1. Which of the following are addressed during the initial prenatal visit and examination?
   a. Genetic diseases/conditions in the family
   b. Kidney and heart diseases/conditions and diabetes
   c. Nutritional deficiencies
   d. All of the above

2. Which of the following is the medical term for the period of development from conception to birth?
   a. Parturition
   b. Postcoital
   c. Prenatal
   d. Puerperium
   e. Postnatal

3. What is the appropriate medical term to describe implantation of a fertilized ovum outside of the uterus?
   a. Placenta abruption
   b. Coupling agent
   c. Ectopic pregnancy
   d. Gestational diabetes

4. The Pap smear is designed to detect which type of cancer?
   a. Cervical
   b. Vaginal
   c. Ovarian
   d. Both a and b
   e. All of the above

5. Which of the following terms describes the procedure where cells are destroyed by an electrical current?
   a. Fulguration
   b. Cryosurgery
   c. Colposcopy
   d. Dysplasia

6. Which of the following symptoms might indicate an ectopic pregnancy?
   a. One-sided abdominal or pelvic pain
   b. Fever
   c. Infertility
   d. Blood-tinged mucous vaginal discharge
   e. Negative pregnancy test

7. Which of the following is the term given to a woman who has not carried a pregnancy to birth?
   a. Nullipara
   b. Primigravida
   c. Multigravida
   d. Gravidity

8. Which of the following might be included in post–IUD insertion patient education?
   a. It is possible to become pregnant with an IUD in place.
   b. No bleeding is expected other than regular menstruation.
   c. The IUD is excellent protection against STDs.
   d. An IUD must be replaced every year.
   e. Cramping after IUD insertion rarely occurs.

9. The small flexible ring that is inserted in the vagina and slowly releases hormones is called what?
   a. A diaphragm
   b. A cervical cap
   c. Spermicide
   d. A vaginal ring

10. During a prenatal visit, the urine is tested for which two substances?
   a. Drugs, including alcohol, and glucose
   b. Infection and glucose
   c. Glucose and protein
   d. Bilirubin and protein
   e. Nitrates and urobilinogen

LEARNING APPLICATION

Critical Thinking

1. Calculate an expected date of confinement (EDC) using Nägele's rule. The patient's first day of her last monthly period (LMP) was April 20, 2017.

   EDC: ______________________________

2. A pregnant woman, who has had no prenatal care, has not had a period for 6 months. She has called the OB/GYN clinic to schedule an appointment because she is experiencing vaginal bleeding. She continues to feel fetal movement.
   a. What laboratory tests or procedures will the provider order?

   ____

   ____

   b. What might you say to the patient to reassure her during this stressful time?

   ____

   ____

3. Lower abdominal pain and back pain that increases just before and during menses may be caused by what condition? With your knowledge of this condition, what might the provider order for treatment of this condition and why?

   ____

   ____

   ____

   ____

   ____

4. Emily Harris is scheduled to have a cervical punch biopsy. What is the primary reason for a cervical punch biopsy? Explain the postbiopsy instructions she will need.

5. A 17-year-old girl has missed her period and has called the clinic describing sharp, right lower quadrant pain. What procedures will assist the provider in making a diagnosis?

Case Studies

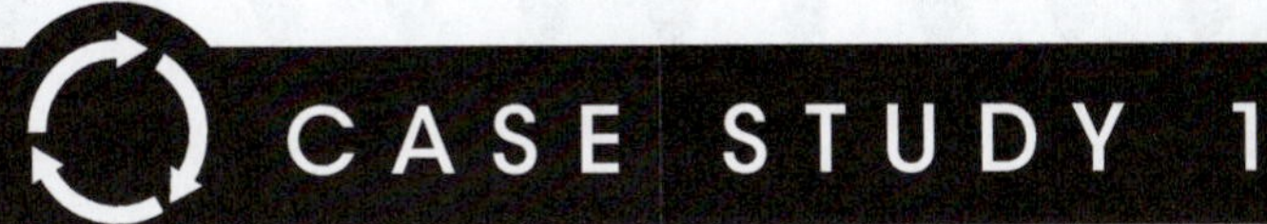

In the clinic, the provider instructs you that a Pap smear and pelvic examination will be performed on Ms. Dobson in Room 1.

CASE STUDY REVIEW QUESTION

1. Describe your role in assisting with these procedures.

Research Activity

Access a Web site for expectant parents to locate information about the following:

- Create fact sheets about each trimester to utilize for patient education.
- Create an outline of tests that are commonly performed during pregnancy in order to address a patient's possible concerns.

ATTRIBUTES OF PROFESSIONALISM

Describe the ways in which you, the medical assistant, can display a calm, professional, and caring manner to a patient during her annual GYN examination. Incorporate the Attributes of Professionalism in your response.

Name ______________________ Date ________ Score ________

CHAPTER 26

Pediatrics

VOCABULARY BUILDER

Misspelled Words

Find the words below that are misspelled; circle them, and then correctly spell them in the spaces provided.

arosolized	exudates	neyonate
circumcision	fontaneles	phynelketonuria
cokelear implantation	myringotomy	

_______________ _______________ _______________

_______________ _______________ _______________

Matching

Match each vocabulary term to its definition.

____ 1. Aerosolized	A. Placement of a tube through the tympanic membrane
____ 2. Exudate	B. Soft spot lying between the bones of the skull of a fetus, newborn, or infant
____ 3. Lyophilized	C. A form of medication that requires reconstitution
____ 4. Myringotomy	D. Incision into the tympanic membrane
____ 5. Neonate	E. Newborn child, typically less than a month old
____ 6. Organomercurial	F. An oozing of pus
____ 7. Phenylketonuria	G. Dispensed by means of a mist
____ 8. Tympanostomy	H. Any organic compound containing mercury
____ 9. Fontanel	I. Hereditary disease that is caused by the body's inability to oxidize the amino acid phenylalanine

LEARNING REVIEW

Short Answer

1. Mary O'Keefe has called for an emergency appointment with Dr. King for her 3-year-old son, Chris, who awakened during the night with a high fever and severe pain in his right ear, which is draining. Gwen Carr, CMA (AAMA), must prepare the examination room for the patient. Based on Chris's symptoms, what equipment will Gwen want to assemble for Dr. King's physical examination of Chris? List the equipment in the order it will most likely be used in the examination.

2. When Mary O'Keefe arrives with her son, Gwen takes them to examination room 2 and prepares the patient for Dr. King's physical examination. Gwen takes and records the child's vital signs: T 102.1°F (Ax); P 115 (AP) bounding, sinus arrhythmia; R 28; BP 76/42 rt. arm, sitting. Gwen tells Mary that Dr. King will be examining Chris's ear and may want to take some laboratory tests.

   A. What method should Gwen use to take Chris's temperature?

   B. What method should Gwen use to measure Chris's pulse? Where on the body is this measured?

   C. Are Chris's vital signs normal?

   D. Chris is fussy and disagreeable, but not uncooperative, while Gwen takes his vital signs. What can a medical assistant do to facilitate the measurement of a fussy child's vital signs?

3. Gwen assists Dr. King with the physical examination of the patient. After assessing the vital sign measurements taken by the medical assistant, Dr. King examines Chris's ear and lungs. A swab of fluid discharge is taken from the patient's ear. What is the role of the medical assistant during the provider's examination of this patient?

4. Dr. King makes a clinical diagnosis of otitis media for this patient and orders laboratory testing to be performed on the patient's specimen. What criteria are necessary for a provider to make a clinical diagnosis?

____

____

____

____

5. What is otitis media? Why are children more at risk for this condition? How is otitis media commonly treated? What patient education can the health care team offer? (Consult a medical reference or encyclopedia for help in answering this question.)

____

____

____

____

____

____

____

____

CERTIFICATION REVIEW

These questions are designed to mimic the certification examination. Select the best response.

1. What is a common illness during childhood that has a primary symptom of a "bark-like" cough?
   a. Tonsillitis
   b. Pediculosis
   c. Croup
   d. Asthma
2. A 1-year-old child should have a respiratory rate in what range?
   a. 20 to 30 breaths per minute
   b. 20 to 40 breaths per minute
   c. 16 to 20 breaths per minute
   d. 12 to 20 breaths per minute
   e. 8 to 16 breaths per minute
3. What is otitis media?
   a. An inflammation of the middle ear
   b. An infestation of parasitic lice
   c. A spasm of the bronchi
   d. An infection of the tonsils

4. When administering a vaccine to a pediatric patient, which of the following would be appropriate needle gauges?
   a. 8- to 10-gauge needle
   b. 14- to 16-gauge needle
   c. 18- to 20-gauge needle
   d. 22- to 25-gauge needle
   e. 27- to 29-gauge needle
5. What is the preferred site for injections for a child younger than 2 years old?
   a. The vastus lateralis
   b. The gluteus medius
   c. The deltoid
   d. Any of the above is acceptable
6. The infant stage of development begins and ends at what ages?
   a. Birth to 1 month
   b. 2 months to 6 months
   c. 6 months to 1 year
   d. Birth to 3 months
   e. 1 month to 1 year
7. When administering vaccines, what should be taken into consideration to ensure optimal response?
   a. Proper needle selection
   b. Reconstitution
   c. Inspecting the vaccine
   d. All of the above
8. For most infants requiring an intramuscular injection, which of the following needles is most appropriate?
   a. ¾-inch 27-gauge needle
   b. 1-inch 22-gauge needle
   c. 1½-inch 20-gauge needle
   d. 1-inch 16-gauge needle
   e. Any of the above
9. Which of the following immunizations should be given subcutaneously?
   a. Varicella
   b. MMR
   c. HPV
   d. Both a and b
10. Length and weight of an infant are plotted on which document?
   a. Medication record
   b. Demographic record
   c. Growth chart
   d. Lab results
   e. All of the above

LEARNING APPLICATION

Critical Thinking

1. You notice when you undress a 2-year-old child to prepare for a physical examination that there are bruises on the buttocks and what appear to be burns on the feet. What course of action do you take?

2. Explain the importance of growth charts.

3. Describe the appropriate positions in which to place an infant for obtaining a rectal temperature.

4. Describe the appearance of the pediatric urine collection bag. What is the best way to make certain it will adhere to the child's body?

5. Explain the type of chart used to test visual acuity in young children.

6. What do the curved lines printed across growth charts indicate?

7. Arleigh Mountjoy is in the office for her 12-month checkup. She is up to date on all of her immunizations. Refer to the recommended immunization schedule on page 689 of the text and list the immunizations that should be given at this visit.

8. Your provider has asked you to plot Arleigh and her twin brother Aaron's growth on a growth chart. See page 704 in your text and determine their growth percentile ranking for both height and weight based on the following information:

   Arleigh: Weight 20 lbs, Length 30 inches

   Aaron: Weight 27 lbs, Length 31 inches

   Arleigh growth percentiles: ____ Weight, ____ Length

   Aaron growth percentiles: ____ Weight, ____ Length

Case Studies

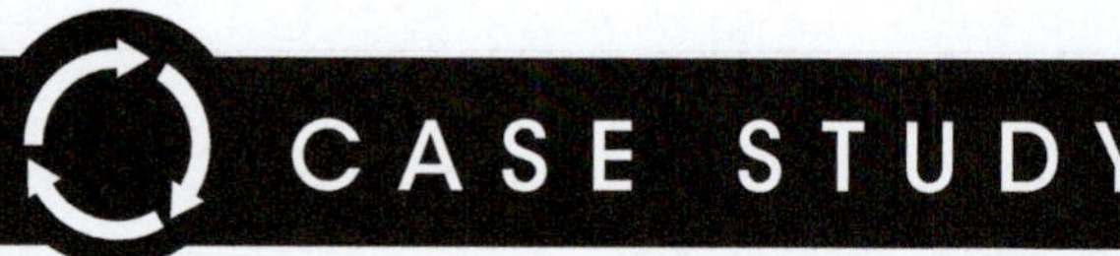

CASE STUDY 1

The following is a true story of a young boy (about 8 years of age) who came into the office with testicular torsion, which occurs when the testicle twists on its cord and often becomes ischemic, resulting in tissue death. The surgeon needed to explore the area to determine if the testicle could be saved or if it needed to be removed. The testicle is usually quite swollen and tender with this condition. When the child was told that he needed to go to the surgery center and that the doctor would take care of his problem and make him feel better, he began to cry. He was inconsolable. Why do you think he was so upset? Here are some options to discuss with classmates:

1. He was afraid of the pain.
2. He was afraid of the surgery.
3. He was embarrassed.
4. Other?

CASE STUDY REVIEW QUESTION

1. Discuss what you could do as a medical assistant to help the boy and his parents with the above scenario. The reason the child was afraid might surprise you and reminds us all to be careful not to assume we know what a patient is thinking.

   ____

   ____

ATTRIBUTES OF PROFESSIONALISM

As you respond to the following question, think of how your experiences will affect how you treat your patients.

1. Think of your first memory of going to a doctor's office or getting any medical treatment. Think of how you felt. You may have more than one vivid memory, or you may have to think to come up with any memories. Maybe your memories are not from a hospital or doctor's office but about medical care received from your parents, grandparents, or a neighbor. Your memories might not be completely accurate because they are a child's perception, but the feelings are real. This awareness can help you interact well with your young patients. Try to respect the feelings they have and strive to make them comfortable. Reassure them as much as you can. Circle all of the words from the following list that came to mind as you completed this exercise

(if you have more than one incident to remember, use different colored inks to circle the words). You may even add a couple of your own descriptors if necessary.

helpless	pain	invaded
embarrassed	guilt	angry
alone	afraid of being punished	afraid of what was happening
afraid of pain	happy with the attention	dizzy
relieved	loved	powerless
excited	safe	afraid of the blood
stupid	other: ______________	other: ______________

2. Which of the Attributes of Professionalism might assist you when caring for your pediatric patient?

____
____
____
____
____
____
____
____
____
____
____

Name ____________________ Date ________ Score ________

CHAPTER 27

Male Reproductive System

VOCABULARY BUILDER

Misspelled Words

Find the words below that are misspelled; circle them, and then correctly spell them in the space provided.

balanitis	nocturia	retension
criptorchidism	orchiecktomy	spermatogenesis
lybido	phymosis	

____________	____________	____________
____________	____________	____________

Matching

Match each term in column I to its description in column II.

	Column I	Column II
____	1. Cryptorchidism	A. Sexual drive
____	2. Intravenous pyelogram	B. Urine held in the bladder; inability to empty the bladder
____	3. Orchiectomy	C. Swelling and/or inflammation of the glans penis
____	4. Hypogonadism	D. Undescended testicle
____	5. Retention	E. X-ray study of the kidneys, ureter, and bladder using a contrast medium
____	6. Transurethral resection	F. A prolonged erection lasting more than 4 hours that may occur with or without sexual stimulation
____	7. Balanitis	G. A benign enlargement of the prostate
____	8. BPH	H. Removal of prostate tissue using a device inserted through the urethra
____	9. Libido	I. Surgical excision of a testicle
____	10. Priapism	J. Syndrome where the testes produce little or no testosterone

LEARNING REVIEW

Short Answer

1. Using the textbook, a medical dictionary, or the Internet to assist you, list at least one common disorder that would adversely affect each part of the male reproduction anatomy listed below.

Part	Common Disorder(s)
1. Epididymis	______________________
2. Testicle	______________________
3. Urinary bladder	______________________
4. Prostate gland	______________________
5. Urethra	______________________
6. Glans penis	______________________

2. List at least two symptoms of a benign hypertrophic prostate gland.

____

____

3. The third leading cause of cancer deaths among men is ______________.

4. Name at least two sexually transmitted diseases.

____

5. PSA tests should be performed ______________ beginning at age 40.

CERTIFICATION REVIEW

These questions are designed to mimic the certification examination. Select the best response.

1. TURP is the abbreviation for what medical procedure?
   a. Transurethral resuscitation of the prostate
   b. Transurethral resection of the prostate
   c. Therapeutic resection of the prostate
   d. Transurethral reattachment of the prostate

2. How often should a male examine the testicles after the onset of puberty?
   a. Every 6 months
   b. Once a year
   c. Every month
   d. Every 3 months
   e. Biannually

3. What does a urodynamic study evaluate?
   a. Bladder capacity
   b. Strength of contraction
   c. The ability to retain urine
   d. All of the above

4. Which of the following causes balanitis?
   a. Bacteria
   b. Fungi
   c. Soap
   d. Injury
   e. All of the above

5. Which of the following is *not* a sexually transmitted disease (STD) that afflicts men?
   a. Genital herpes
   b. Chlamydia
   c. Gonorrhea
   d. Epididymis

6. Which of the following STDs is *not* treated with antibiotics?
   a. Chlamydia infection
   b. Gonorrhea
   c. Syphilis
   d. Genital herpes
   e. None of the above

7. Which of the following is a treatment for erectile dysfunction?
   a. Oral medications
   b. Localized injected medications
   c. Penile implant
   d. All of the above

8. Gonorrhea is diagnosed by what laboratory test?
   a. Urinalysis
   b. Urethral smear
   c. Culture of lesion
   d. Blood test
   e. KOH prep

9. Which of the following is a predisposing factor for testicular cancer?
   a. Cryptorchidism
   b. STDs
   c. History of mumps
   d. Both a and c

10. What is the medical term for inflammation of the prostate?
    a. Prostatitis
    b. Epididymitis
    c. Balanitis
    d. Urethritis
    e. Prostatectomy

LEARNING APPLICATION

Critical Thinking

1. Describe how a testicular self-examination should be performed.

2. What is the purpose of severing the vas deferens?

3. List several symptoms of BPH and explain why the symptoms occur.

4. Describe the blood test that is helpful in the diagnosis of prostatic cancer.

5. At what PSA level does the provider consider the possibility that the patient may have cancer of the prostate?

6. Explain why BPH is more common in men aged 50 years and older.

7. What age group is afflicted by testicular cancer, and how can the patient take action to detect it?

8. How is a rectal examination on a patient useful to the provider in determining a diagnosis for a patient who has nocturia?

Case Studies

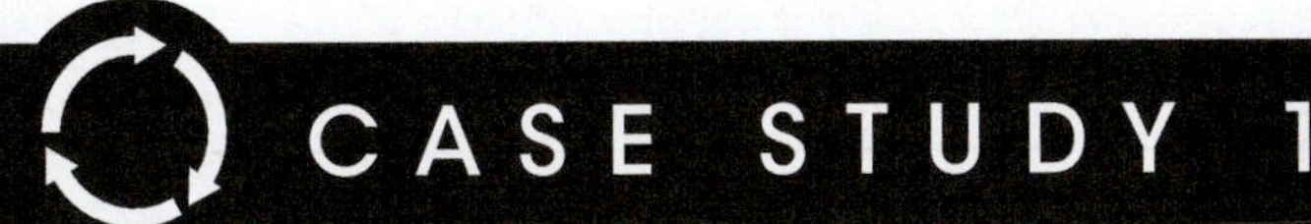

CASE STUDY REVIEW QUESTION

1. Mr. Jones, a 75-year-old patient, has just been diagnosed with prostatic cancer. The provider has explained what is to be expected, but Mr. Jones is upset and asks you for your help in understanding the disease and treatment. How will you help him?

Role-Play Exercise

Research the latest recommendations for testicular-self exam from sites such as www.testicularcancersociety.org and www.cancer.org. Print the instructions for teaching testicular self-exam. Select a partner, and using the testicular self-exam guidelines, practice teaching the correct method of testicular exam to your patient (partner) and then switch roles.

ATTRIBUTES OF PROFESSIONALISM

How do you think you will feel when assisting with a genitourinary examination or procedure on a male patient? Do you think it will be easier if the patient is much younger or much older than you are? Do you think older medical assistants feel more comfortable assisting with these types of examinations, regardless of their professional experience? Do you think you will become more comfortable with time? Do you think your male patient is also uncomfortable? After giving these questions some thought, answer the following questions. Discuss your ideas with other students. Discuss your ideas with male friends, family members, or classmates to gain more perspectives.

1. Do you think your behavior or attitude will have anything to do with your patient's comfort level?

2. In what ways can you display the Attributes of Professionalism during a male genitourinary examination/procedure?

3. In what ways could you assist your patient to become more comfortable?

Name ____________________ Date ________ Score ________

CHAPTER 28

Gerontology

VOCABULARY BUILDER

Misspelled Words and Definitions

Find the words in Column I below that are misspelled; circle them, and correctly spell them in the space provided. Then match each vocabulary term in Column I with the corresponding definition listed in Column II.

	Column I	Correct Spelling	Column II
____	1. Arterialsclerosis	____________	A. The branch of medicine that is concerned with the problems of older adults
____	2. Demenetia	____________	B. Disease marked by degeneration of the macular area of the retina of the eye
____	3. Geriatrics	____________	C. Progressive loss of hearing ability caused by the normal aging process
____	4. Incontinance	____________	D. Temporary loss of blood to the brain, causing stroke-like symptoms
____	5. Macular degeneration	____________	E. Urine remaining in the bladder after urination
____	6. Pernicous anemia	____________	F. Loss of the ability to retain urine in the bladder
____	7. Presbycusis	____________	G. Disorder involving the stomach that causes a deficiency of red blood cells
____	8. Residule urine	____________	H. Decrease in cognitive abilities, especially memory impairment, often associated with Alzheimer and Parkinson diseases
____	9. Transiant ischemic attack	____________	I. Disease that leads to thickening, hardening, and loss of elasticity of the arteries

LEARNING REVIEW

Short Answer

1. List at least five ways to improve communication with the geriatric patient who has memory impairment.

2. Why is gerontology becoming more recognized?

3. Why does food become less appealing as one ages, often decreasing the desire to eat and causing weight loss?

4. Fill in the chart below, listing two problems that might occur with each system as people age. The first row has been filled out as an example for you.

A. Vision and hearing

B. Taste and smell

C. Integumentary system

D. Nervous system

E. Musculoskeletal system

F. Respiratory system

G. Cardiovascular system

H. Gastrointestinal system

I. Urinary system

J. Reproductive system

CERTIFICATION REVIEW

These questions are designed to mimic the certification examination. Select the best response.

1. Dementia can include which of the following symptoms?
   a. Memory loss
   b. Confusion
   c. Depression and agitation
   d. All of the above

2. The nervous system is affected by aging, resulting in all of the following symptoms except what?
   a. Insomnia
   b. Problems with balance
   c. Increased pain sensation
   d. Problems with temperature regulation
   e. Increased visual acuity

3. The buildup of plaque in blood vessels is called what?
   a. Incontinence
   b. Heart attack
   c. Arteriosclerosis
   d. Cardiopulmonary dysfunction

4. What is the name for the progressive loss of hearing ability caused by the normal aging process?
   a. Senility
   b. Presbycusis
   c. Deafness
   d. Audio deficiency
   e. Muted sound recognition

5. Poor nutrition and poor absorption of nutrients can result in what?
   a. Anemia
   b. Malnutrition
   c. Weight gain
   d. Both a and b

6. Which of the following is a way to ensure that an adult with hearing impairment is able to understand instructions?
   a. Providing written instructions
   b. Facing the adult with hearing impairment when speaking
   c. Ensuring that the environment is quiet without distractions
   d. Including a patient's support system
   e. All of the above

7. Loss of a spouse, chronic illness, and financial difficulties can cause which of the following in older adults?
   a. Dementia
   b. Depression
   c. Myocardial infarction
   d. Arteriosclerosis

8. Changes in an area of the retina that is associated with aging is called what?
   a. Macular degeneration
   b. Glaucoma
   c. Cataracts
   d. Conjunctivitis
   e. All of the above

9. An unusually high body temperature is termed what?
   a. Hypothermia
   b. Hyperthermia
   c. Hyperemesis
   d. Hypochondria

10. Being aware of feelings, emotions, and behavior of another is considered what?
   a. Sympathy
   b. Empathy
   c. Dystrophy
   d. Depression
   e. Projection

LEARNING APPLICATION

Critical Thinking

1. What are some ways that older adults can keep their bones from becoming brittle?

2. Describe a vision problem that leaves older adults with difficulty seeing color intensity.

3. What are four causes of urinary incontinence?

4. List three ways to enhance communication with older adults.

5. What is the best way to approach a person with visual impairment?

6. How can you encourage older adults to choose a healthy lifestyle?

7. What are some strategies for older adults to keep mentally and physically stimulated?

8. Describe strategies for communicating with patients who have hearing impairments.

Case Studies

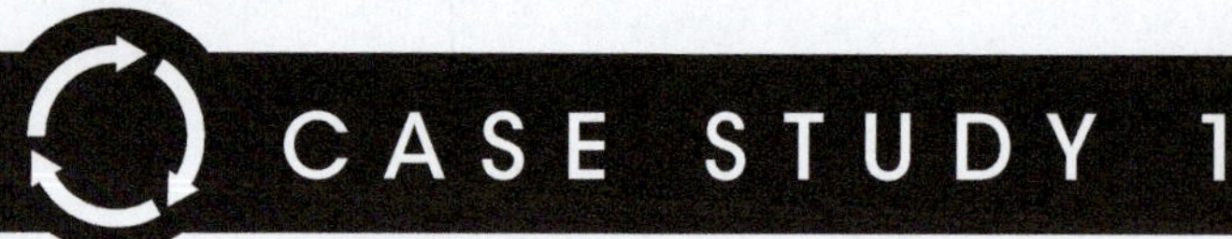

CASE STUDY 1

Sam Jones, 84 years old, has been examined by the provider and is ready to leave the clinic. Mr. Jones tells you that he has trouble remembering to take the many medications the doctor has given him.

CASE STUDY REVIEW QUESTION

1. As a medical assistant, what can you do to help Sam remember to take his medication?

____

____

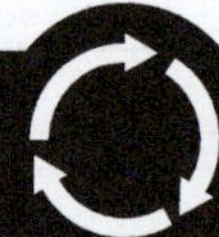

CASE STUDY 2

Adelaide Robinson, 83 years old, has an appointment Thursday morning for a recheck of her most recent complaint. She tells you that she is moving slower than she did just 6 months ago, and she has noticed less flexibility as well.

CASE STUDY REVIEW QUESTIONS

1. What are the possible causes of Mrs. Robinson's complaints?

____

____

____

____

2. What effect could these problems have on Mrs. Robinson's daily routine?

____

____

3. What might Dr. King suggest Mrs. Robinson do to help alleviate her symptoms?

____

____

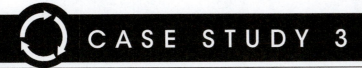

Sally Donovan, 92 years old, is in the gerontology clinic today. Her main concern, problem, and reason for appointment is that she "cannot taste or smell much anymore and food doesn't taste good." She wants suggestions from the provider about how to improve her senses of taste and smell so she can enjoy food more freely.

CASE STUDY REVIEW QUESTIONS

1. What are some reasons that older adults lose their sense of taste and smell?

2. Describe dangers that can be associated with loss of taste and smell.

ATTRIBUTES OF PROFESSIONALISM

Often, older adults are isolated from their peers and are lonely. A trip to your clinic might be a great chance for the older patient to engage in conversation and have some interaction with other adults. With the understanding that your daily schedule allows only a few minutes for each patient, how can you utilize the Attributes of Professionalism to demonstrate respect for patients while keeping them on task during the history and exam?

Name ______________________ Date __________ Score __________

CHAPTER 29

Examinations and Procedures of Body Systems

VOCABULARY BUILDER

Misspelled Words

Find the words below that are misspelled; circle them, and correctly spell them in the spaces provided. Then fill in the blanks in the sentences that follow with the correct vocabulary terms.

afasia	carbncle	epystaxis
auricle	conjunctyvitis	erythemia
biopsy	demyelination	malaise
bullemia	dislocation	strabismus

______________ ______________ ______________

______________ ______________ ______________

1. A ______________ is an inflammation of the skin and deeper tissues that terminates in slough and suppuration.
2. ______________ is a form of macula showing diffused redness of the skin.
3. Infection of the membranes lining the eyelids is called ______________.
4. Destruction or removal of the myelin sheath is ______________.
5. The provider obtains a representative tissue sample for microscopic examination during a ______________.
6. The medical term for a nosebleed is ______________.
7. A disease that is characterized by binging on food and then vomiting or using laxatives to prevent weight gain is ______________.
8. ______________ is the absence or impairment of the ability to communicate through speech.
9. A general feeling of discomfort or unease is known as ______________.

10. The ________________ is the portion of the external ear that is not directly connected to the head.

11. Joint trauma that involves the ________________ of the head of a bone from its socket is a common injury to the shoulder.

12. ________________ is a disorder in which the eyes do not line up in the same direction.

LEARNING REVIEW

Short Answer

1. List five components of a urinalysis.

2. List two causes of erosion of the mucous lining of the stomach.

3. There are many diseases that can be diagnosed by evaluating a patient's blood. List four blood tests that are commonly ordered.

4. List at least four endoscopic procedures that require a patient to remain NPO.

5. Describe the difference between internal and external respiration.

6. List and describe the three kinds of allergy skin testing.

7. List the supplies needed to assist the provider to perform a neurologic examination.

___

___

8. Describe the difference between instillation and irrigation.

___

___

Image Labeling

1. Identify the parts of the digestive system.

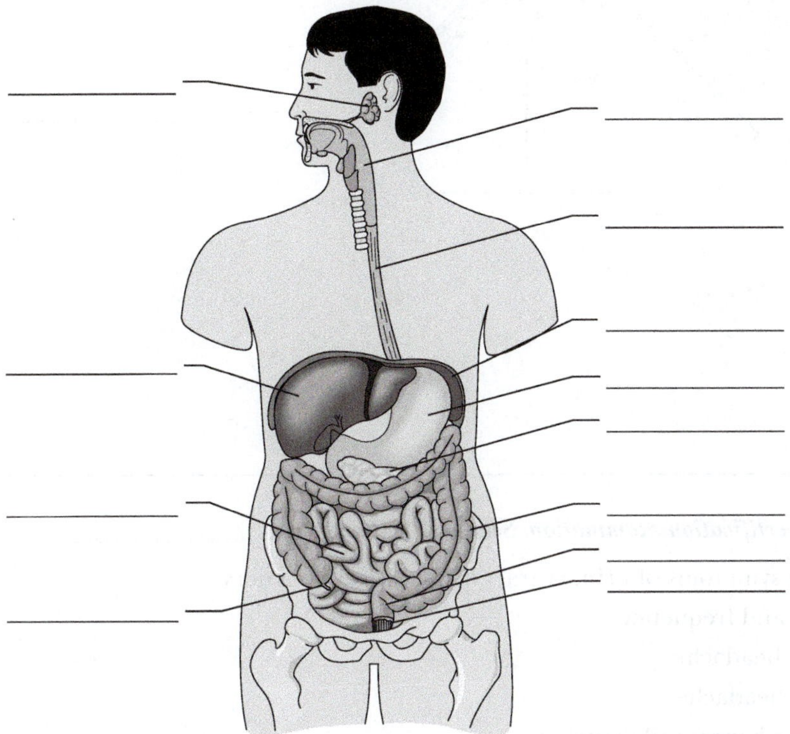

2. Identify the parts of the eye.

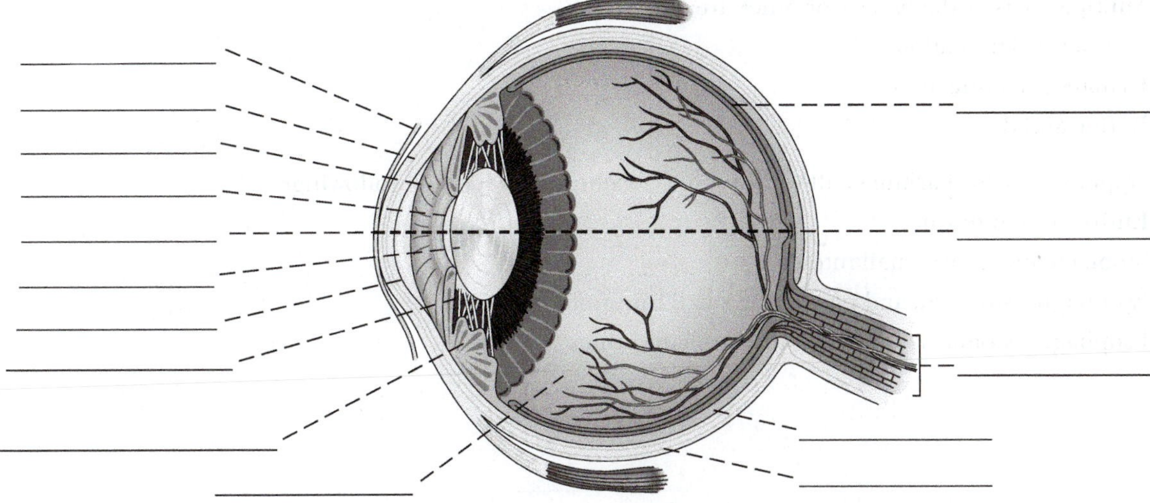

3. Identify the parts of the ear.

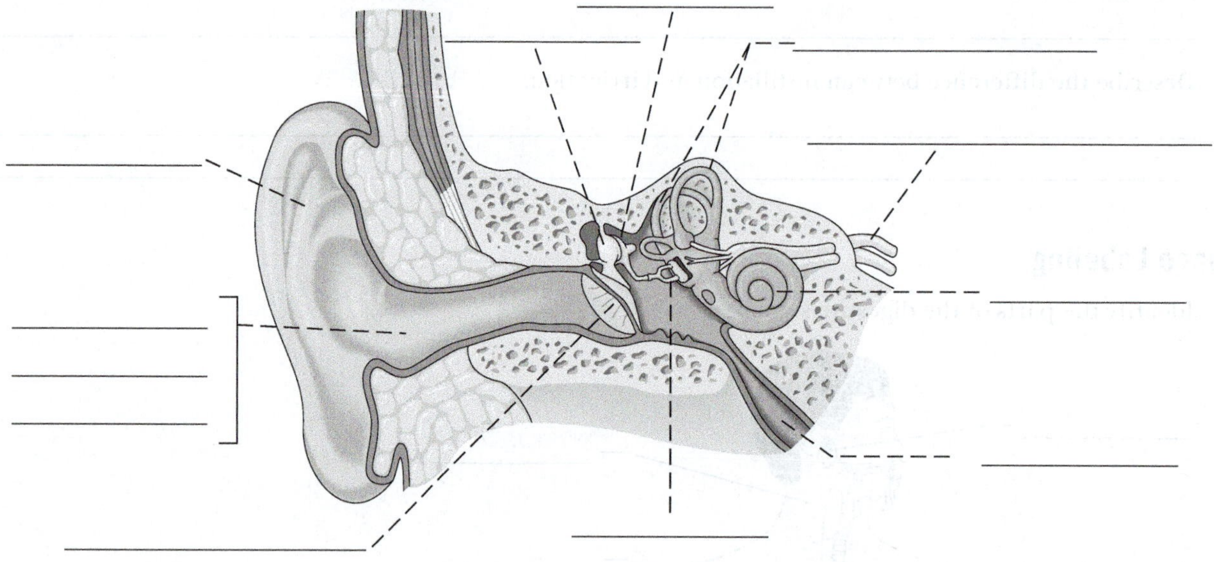

CERTIFICATION REVIEW

These questions are designed to mimic the certification examination. Select the best response.

1. Which of the following are common symptoms of urinary tract diseases and disorders?
   a. Dysuria, proteinuria, hematuria, and frequency
   b. Dysuria, frequency, oliguria, and headache
   c. Hematuria, pain, frequency, and headache
   d. Frequency, hematuria, vaginal discharge, and dysuria

2. Cystitis is another name for what disorder?
   a. Gallbladder disease
   b. Multiple cysts of the breasts or other area
   c. Bladder inflammation
   d. Urinary tract infection
   e. Both c and d

3. An upper GI series (barium swallow) is used to examine which of the following?
   a. Entire large intestine
   b. Stomach and entire small intestine
   c. Esophagus, stomach, and part of the small intestine
   d. Esophagus, stomach, and small and large intestines

4. Which of the following is an eating disorder?
   a. Bulimia
   b. Anorexia nervosa
   c. Diverticulosis
   d. Crohn disease
   e. Both a and b

5. Which of the following charts are used to check for color vision?
   a. Snellen
   b. Ishihara
   c. Landolt C
   d. LEA symbol

6. What is the medical term for increased intraocular pressure?
   a. Glaucoma
   b. Retinal detachment
   c. Cataract
   d. Macular degeneration
   e. Diabetic retinopathy

7. Which of the following is the clear tissue covering the pupil and iris?
   a. Sclera
   b. Lens
   c. Cornea
   d. Retina

8. Which of the following is a simple tool to assess hearing that is commonly used in a provider's office?
   a. Audiometer
   b. Phonograph
   c. Tuning fork
   d. Tympanometer
   e. Both c and d

9. A cholecystectogram is a test to diagnose which of the following?
   a. Kidney stones
   b. Diseases of the gallbladder
   c. Diseases of the blood vessels
   d. Gastrointestinal disorders

10. Which of the following is *not* determined by a chest radiograph?
    a. Bronchitis
    b. Pneumonia
    c. Pharyngitis
    d. Tuberculosis
    e. Lymphedema

LEARNING APPLICATION

Critical Thinking

1. Is there an advantage to catheterizing a patient to obtain a specimen for urinalysis and culture and sensitivity? Why or why not?

2. What is the use and purpose of the audiometer? How is the test administered?

3. Explain the rationale when doing an eye irrigation for flowing solution from the inside canthus to the outer canthus of the eye.

4. Differentiate among bronchitis, emphysema, and asthma.

5. What is the medical assistant's role when assisting with spirometry?

6. What cast care guidelines does the medical assistant give to the patient?

7. When a mental status examination is given, what five areas are being assessed?

8. Explain the medical assistant's role when assisting with a lumbar puncture.

Case Studies

CASE STUDY 1

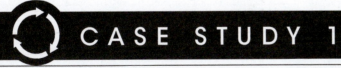

While visiting with family members, your elderly aunt shares with you that she has noticed that her stools are black. This has been happening off and on for several months and now she says her "belly feels swollen" and she is constipated a lot, which is not normal for her.

CASE STUDY REVIEW QUESTIONS

1. How will you respond?

2. Your aunt becomes alarmed and says she is afraid of what they will do to her; maybe she will need surgery, and she cannot leave her husband alone, and what if it is cancer. She obviously has many concerns and is quite worried. How can you assist her?

Role-Play Exercise

Choose a partner and practice educating a patient regarding correctly obtaining stool specimens to screen for occult blood in stool.

1. Make a list of the supplies that will be provided to the patient.

2. Educate your partner regarding the steps to obtain the stool for occult blood testing.

ATTRIBUTES OF PROFESSIONALISM

1. Think of a time when you or a close family member had to go to the provider's office and then go through a diagnostic procedure or test for a medical disorder or disease. List the Attributes of Professionalism that might have been applicable for the medical assistant during this visit.

____

____

____

____

____

____

2. What were some of the feelings that you had during the process? List two or three.

____

____

____

3. How will your experience influence your interaction with your patients when you are assisting with a diagnostic test or procedure? What will you pay special attention to that you might not have if you had not had the experience described above?

____

____

____

Name ______________________ Date ________ Score ________

CHAPTER 30

Assisting with Minor Surgery

VOCABULARY BUILDER

Misspelled Words

Find the words in Column I that are misspelled; circle them, and correctly spell them in the spaces provided. Then match each vocabulary term below with the correct definition in Column II.

	Column I	Correct Spelling	Column II
____	1. Inflamation	____________	A. The trade name for povidone-iodine, a topical anti-infective
____	2. Ephinephrine	____________	B. Partial or complete loss of sensation, with or without loss of consciousness
____	3. Fenestrated	____________	C. Easily broken or torn
____	4. Ligature	____________	D. A hormone secreted by the adrenal medulla in response to stimulation of the sympathetic nervous system; used in conjunction with a local anesthetic; constricts blood vessels to help lessen bleeding during ambulatory surgery
____	5. Hibeclens	____________	E. A condition free from germs, infection, and any form of life
____	6. Anestesia	____________	F. A narrowing or constriction of the lumen of a tube, duct, or hollow organ
____	7. Friable	____________	G. Having an opening, as in a surgical drape
____	8. Betadine	____________	H. Trade name for chlorhexidine gluconate, a topical antiseptic
____	9. Volatile	____________	I. Easily evaporated
____	10. Isopryl alcohol	____________	J. A thread or wire for tying a blood vessel or other structure to constrict or fasten it

_____ 11. Strictures _______________ K. The nonspecific immune response that occurs in reaction to any type of bodily injury

_____ 12. Surgical asepsis _______________ L. A clean, flammable liquid used in medical preparations for external use

Definitions

Match each vocabulary word below with the correct definition.

_____ 1. Approximate

_____ 2. Cautery

_____ 3. Contamination

_____ 4. Infection

_____ 5. Informed consent

_____ 6. Mayo stand/instrument tray

_____ 7. Ratchets

_____ 8. Suture

_____ 9. Swaged/atraumatic

A. To bring together the edges of a wound

B. A surgical needle is attached to a length of suture material

C. Surgical material or thread; may describe the act of sewing with the surgical material and needle

D. An invasion of pathogens into living tissue

E. A voluntary agreement to have a procedure or surgery after a patient has been informed about the risks and benefits

F. A portable metal tray table used for setting up a sterile field for minor surgery and procedures

G. The locking mechanisms on the handles of many surgical instruments

H. The destruction of tissue by burning

I. To make something unclean, often used to describe a sterile area being made "unsterile" or exposing a clean area to a pathogenic substance

LEARNING REVIEW

Short Answer

1. Identify each entry below as an example that follows strict sterile principles or in which the sterile area, field, or tray is contaminated. Write *sterile* or *contaminated* in the spaces provided. If the entry is *contaminated*, write what was done to render it contaminated.

   A. Joe Guerrero, CMA (AAMA), collects used instruments handed to him by Dr. Angie Osborne during a minor surgical procedure to excise an infected sebaceous cyst by placing the instruments in a separate container or area out of view of the patient.

   ____

B. Gwen Carr, CMA (AAMA), sets up a sterile field for a minor surgical procedure. After setting up the field, she remembers that a sterile solution is required and leaves the room to obtain the solution to be poured into a sterile cup.

C. Nancy McFarland, RMA (AMT), removes a dressing from a wound on a patient's arm and then reaches over the sterile field to discard the used dressing in a biohazard waste container that she has placed on the other side of the sterile field that she set up for the procedure.

D. Patient Edith Leonard will not stop talking and asking questions as Liz Corbin, CMA (AAMA), removes sutures from a small wound on Edith's arm that was sustained during a recent fall. The medical assistant is careful to time her responses to Edith so that she is not talking when she is working directly over the sterile field.

E. Thomas Myers, CCMA (NHA), applies sterile gloves in preparation to assist Dr. Lewis with a minor surgical procedure. During the procedure, he comforts the patient and assists the provider as required. When Thomas's hands are not in use, he keeps them down at his sides, careful not to touch his gloved hands to his clothing or any other nonsterile item.

2. Living tissue surfaces, such as skin, cannot be sterilized. Name two examples of ways that skin can be rid of as many pathogens as possible before the use of a sterile covering.

3. Identify and describe the most widely used method of sterilization in the ambulatory care setting.

4. List six general rules that ensure proper sterilization when using an autoclave.

5. Identify the recommended requirements for effective sterilization in an autoclave.

Temperature ____________________

Time for sterilization of unwrapped items ____________________

Time for sterilization of loosely wrapped items ____________________

Time for sterilization of tightly wrapped items ____________________

Frequency of draining of water and cleaning of autoclave ____________________

MATCHING I

Match the following equipment with the correct aseptic method. For each instrument or item below, identify the method used for proper asepsis: chemical disinfection (CD), chemical sterilization (CS), or steam sterilization (SS) in an autoclave.

_______ 1. Percussion hammer

_______ 2. Wrapped surgical instruments

_______ 3. Stethoscopes

_______ 4. Fiber optic endoscopes

_______ 5. Countertops

_______ 6. Wheelchairs

_______ 7. Gynecologic instruments

_______ 8. Examination tables

MATCHING II

Identify each action that follows as an action appropriate to medical aseptic hand washing technique (MAH) or surgical aseptic hand washing technique (SAH).

_______ 1. Do not apply lotion.

_______ 2. Glove for sterility.

_______ 3. One-minute duration

_______ 4. Hold hands up during washing and rinsing.

_______ 5. Apply lotion.

_______ 6. Wash hands, wrists, and forearms to the elbows.

_______ 7. Hold hands down during rinsing.

_______ 8. Three- to 6-minute duration

CERTIFICATION REVIEW

These questions are designed to mimic the certification examination. Select the best response.

1. What is the term for surgical instruments that have opposing cutting edges?
   a. Hemostats
   b. Probes
   c. Scissors
   d. Scalpels
2. What is the purpose of surgical instruments that have ratchets?
   a. Cutting
   b. Clamping
   c. Probing
   d. Exploring
   e. Opening
3. Which of the following is not a method of sterilization?
   a. Boiling sterilization
   b. Gas sterilization
   c. Steam sterilization
   d. Dry heat sterilization
4. What is the term for an item that is free from all microorganisms and their spores?
   a. Contaminated
   b. Sterile
   c. Decontaminated
   d. Clean
   e. Cultured
5. An informed consent should include what information?
   a. Risks of the procedure
   b. Alternate therapies
   c. Name and description of the procedure
   d. All of the above
6. How many inches are considered an acceptable border between a sterile and a nonsterile area?
   a. 1
   b. 2
   c. 4
   d. 5
   e. 6 inches
7. The preferred length for suture material, because it is manageable yet long enough to complete most suture procedures, is which of the following lengths?
   a. 10 inches
   b. 8 inches
   c. 12 inches
   d. 18 inches

8. When loading an autoclave, it is important to leave how much space between packages?
   a. 1 to 2 inches
   b. 1 to 3 inches
   c. 2 to 3 inches
   d. 2 to 4 inches
   e. 3 to 5 inches

9. When assisting the provider with a minor surgery, which is the correct order of the activities listed below?
   1. Set up sterile field
   2. Wash hands
   3. Place sterile instruments and supplies on the sterile field
   4. Gather equipment and supplies
      a. 2, 4, 1, 3
      b. 1, 2, 3, 4
      c. 2, 1, 3, 4
      d. 4, 2, 1, 3

10. Which of the following is considered a sterile principle?
    a. A sterile object may not touch a nonsterile object.
    b. Turning your back on a sterile field is allowable.
    c. Reaching over the sterile field is allowable with gloved hands.
    d. Some sterile objects are still considered sterile when wet.
    e. Sterile items are considered sterile as long as they rest at least ½ inch from nonsterile items.

LEARNING APPLICATION

Critical Thinking

1. What is the purpose of OSHA's Bloodborne Pathogen Standard and whom does it cover?

____

____

____

____

____

2. You are setting up a sterile surgical tray and have already applied your sterile gloves before you realize you forgot to place the suture package on the tray. You have several options. What are they, and what are the advantages and disadvantages of each?

____

____

____

____

____

____

____

____

3. What would be the rationale behind leaving a wound open rather than suturing it? On what basis would the provider make the decision?

4. While you are preparing a patient for surgery, he confides in you that he doesn't have anyone to drive him home, but he only lives three miles away and he can drive himself. How do you respond?

5. You have thoroughly explained the postoperative instructions to the patient and caregiver. Are written instructions also necessary? Why or why not?

6. While pouring a sterile solution into a bowl on the sterile field, you accidentally splash a very tiny amount of the solution onto the field. What is your next step? Explain your actions.

7. During an incision and drainage of a localized infection, you notice a large amount of exudate from the side. What precautions should you take?

Case Studies

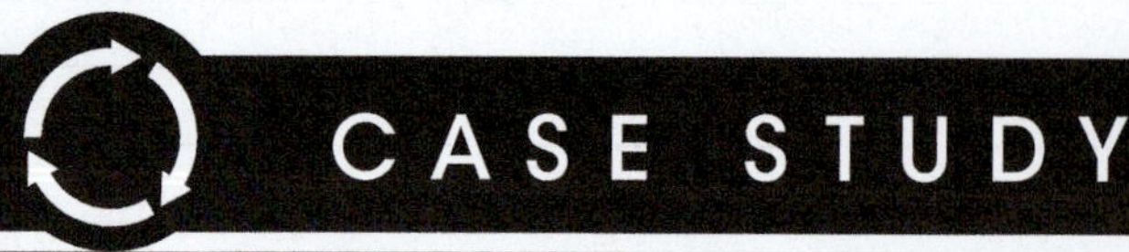

CASE STUDY 1

Gwen Carr, CMA (AAMA), is responsible for maintaining and cleaning the autoclave at Inner City Health Care. Because this equipment is used every day to sterilize instruments, Gwen cleans the inner chamber of the autoclave daily. Once a week, she gives the autoclave a thorough cleaning.

CASE STUDY REVIEW QUESTIONS

1. Describe Gwen's daily cleaning procedure.

2. Describe Gwen's weekly cleaning procedure.

3. Why is proper maintenance and cleaning of the autoclave important?

CASE STUDY 2

Gwen works with a variety of instruments and supplies as she assists in ambulatory care surgery. Answer the following questions related to surgical instruments and supplies.

CASE STUDY REVIEW QUESTIONS

1. From the selection that follows, identify each instrument by name. In the spaces provided, give a brief description of each instrument's use.

Instrument	Instrument Name	Uses

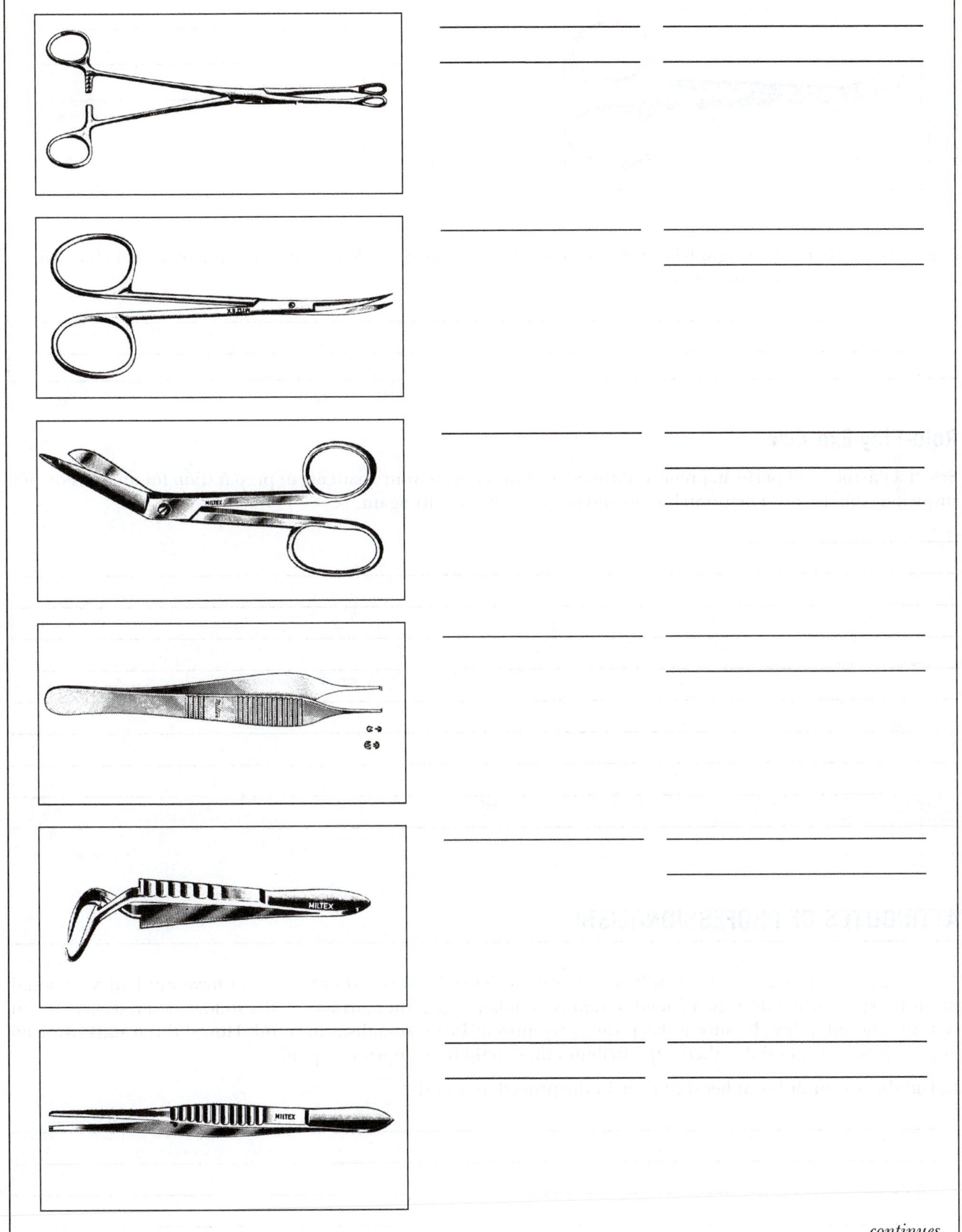

continues

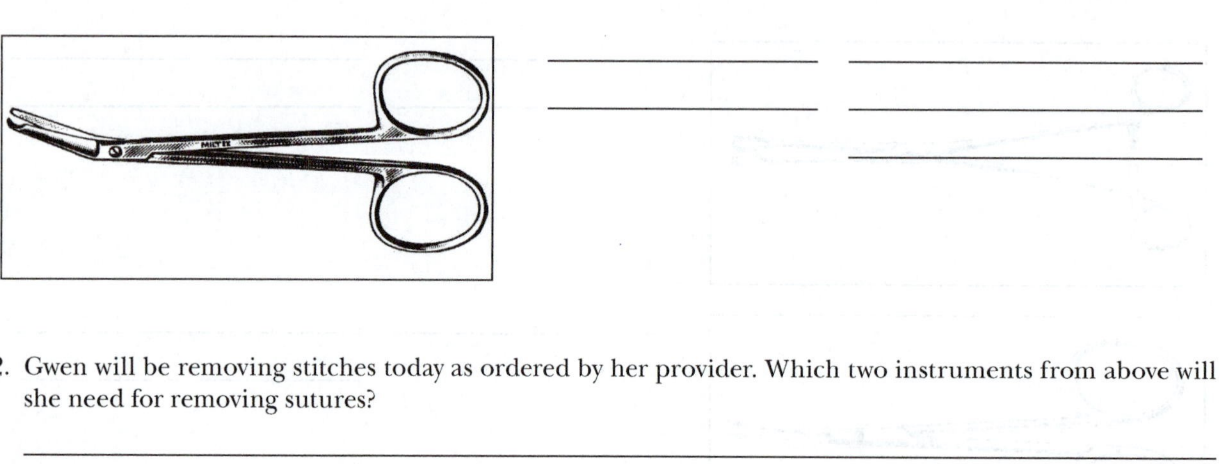

2. Gwen will be removing stitches today as ordered by her provider. Which two instruments from above will she need for removing sutures?

Role-Play Exercise

Select a partner and perform preprocedure education. Educate your "patient" in preparation for an excision of a suspicious skin lesion. Then switch roles and perform the activity again.

ATTRIBUTES OF PROFESSIONALISM

Think of a time when you or a family member experienced a surgical event. If you have not had a personal surgical experience, interview a friend or family member and gather answers to the following questions. As you conduct the interview, be sure to keep the Attributes of Professionalism in mind. How did the staff involved display these attributes? Are there any attributes they could have improved upon?

1. Did the doctor or his or her staff explain the procedure clearly?

2. Were your questions answered to your satisfaction?

3. What was of greatest concern to you (financial concerns, pain, recovery, results, etc.)?

4. What could have made the experience better?

Name ______________________ Date __________ Score __________

CHAPTER 31

Diagnostic Imaging

VOCABULARY BUILDER

Misspelled Words

Find the words below that are misspelled; circle them, and correctly spell them in the spaces provided. Then write the correct vocabulary terms next to the corresponding definitions.

dosimeter	magnetic resonence imaging	radiolusent
echocardiogram	oscilloscope	transducer
floroscope	position emission tomography	
isotopes	radialpaque	

______________ ______________ ______________

______________ ______________ ______________

1. ______________ Use of fluorescent screen that shows images of objects inserted between the tube and the screen
2. ______________ Sound waves emit from its head during ultrasound
3. ______________ A chemical element
4. ______________ A noninvasive procedure where the patient lies inside a cylinder-shaped machine, or an open-bore machine, in which there is an electromagnet
5. ______________ A radiographic procedure using a computer and radioactive substance
6. ______________ Describes a structure that X-rays do not penetrate
7. ______________ Noninvasive diagnostic method that uses ultrasound to visualize internal cardiac structure, including valves
8. ______________ Small, badge-like device worn above the waist which measures the amount of X-rays a person is exposed to
9. ______________ Describes a structure X-rays penetrate easily
10. ______________ An electronic device used for recording electrical activity of the heart, brain, and muscular tissues

Fill in the blank

Complete the sentences using key terms from the chapter.

1. ________________ ultrasonography uses sound waves to explore blood flow through major vessels in the body.
2. A common disorder of the bones that occurs in postmenopausal women is ________________.
3. When a patient is undergoing radiation therapy, they may exhibit signs of ________________, an inflammation and ulceration of the mouth.
4. Patients that experience ________________ may need to be premedicated with an antianxiety agent prior to a scheduled MRI.
5. Depending on a woman's risk factors, a screening ________________ should be obtained between age 40 and 45 years.
6. ________________ is a noninvasive screening tool to measure one's risk for fractures.
7. A vacuum tube generating a focused beam of electrons is known as a ________________ ray tube.
8. A(n) ______________________________ is a device that senses and corrects dangerous cardiac rhythms.
9. Thallium is an example of a ________________.
10. A radionuclide is a ________________ substance that is injected to diagnose diseases such as thyroid disorders.
11. A chest X-ray is an example of a ________________.
12. An MRI is an imaging exam that does not use ________________.
13. Using radiation to shrink the size of a cancerous tumor to reduce pain is considered ________________ care.

LEARNING REVIEW

Short Answer

1. Describe the positions used during X-rays and include the direction of the X-rays, if applicable.

Position	Description	Direction of X-rays
Anteroposterior view (AP)		
Posteroanterior view (PA)		
Lateral view		
Right lateral view (RL)		
Left lateral view (LL)		
Oblique view		
Supine view		
Prone view		

2. For each radiologic test listed below, explain the purpose of the test.

Test	Purpose
Angiography	
Barium swallow (upper GI series)	
Barium enema (lower GI series)	
Cholangiography	
Cholecystography	
Cystography	
Hysterosalpingography	
Intravenous pyelography (IVP)	
Mammography	
Retrograde pyelography	

3. Describe the patient preparation needed for each test: before, during, and after. *NOTE:* Instructions for the following exams may differ depending on the facility and technology involved.

Test	Patient Preparation
Angiography	
Barium swallow (upper GI series)	
Cholangiography	
Cholecystography	
Cystography	
Hysterosalpingography	
Intravenous pyelography (IVP)	
Mammography	
Retrograde pyelography	

4. Why is exposure to radiation dangerous?

____

____

5. What test is performed to study the colon for disease?

____

____

CERTIFICATION REVIEW

These questions are designed to mimic the certification examination. Select the best response.

1. If a patient needs to be NPO before a radiologic procedure and the patient drinks a glass of water 3 hours before the appointment, what must you do?
   a. Water is allowed but nothing else.
   b. The provider must be consulted.
   c. The procedure must be canceled.
   d. Three hours is long enough for the water to be through the patient's system.

2. What are the characteristics of a PET scan?
   a. A radioactive substance is injected into the patient's blood.
   b. Charged particles are given off that combine with particles in the patient's body.
   c. Color images are produced.
   d. Changes in tissues can be detected at a cellular level.
   e. All of the above

3. Which of the following is the definition of palliative?
   a. Relieving symptoms, as well as curing
   b. Curing but not offering much relief of symptoms
   c. Placebo, or an agent that has no effect even though the patient thinks it's helping
   d. Agents, such as pain relievers, used to relieve or alleviate painful or uncomfortable symptoms that do not cure the condition

4. What are the considerations that must be taken into account when storing and safeguarding radiographs?
   a. Radiographs must be protected from light, heat, and moisture
   b. The environment is of little concern; radiographs are basically plastic and can be wiped clean
   c. Radiographs must be kept in a cool, dry place
   d. Humidity has no effect on the films
   e. Both a and c

5. Which is true about medical assistants and their ability to take X-rays?
   a. With additional training, medical assistants can take films of extremities in some states.
   b. If the provider approves, medical assistants can take radiographs as ordered in any state.
   c. Medical assistants must have a basic understanding of radiologic studies for the purpose of patient teaching.
   d. Both a and c

6. Flat plates are known as "plain" films for which of the following reasons?
   a. No contrast medium is used
   b. They require no special technique
   c. They are used only for X-rays of extremities
   d. They do not require the addition of a patient's name
   e. Both a and b

7. In order to obtain an anteroposterior view (AP), which of the following is correct?
   a. The anterior surface of the body faces away from the tube.
   b. The anterior surface of the body faces the tube.
   c. The posterior surface of the body faces the tube.
   d. None of the above

8. MRI and CT scanning are not available for patients with what implantable device?
   a. Metal clips or pins
   b. Pacemaker
   c. Implantable cardioverter-defibrillator
   d. Stainless steel implants
   e. All of the above

9. Stomatitis, bone marrow depression, and nausea and vomiting are side effects of which of the following?
   a. Mammography
   b. Radiation therapy
   c. Gastrography
   d. Infusion therapy

10. Once radiographic films are taken, they become the property of which of the following?
    a. The patient
    b. The provider
    c. The hospital or facility
    d. The insurance company
    e. The radiologist

LEARNING APPLICATION

Critical Thinking

1. Describe the purpose of a lead apron and lead-lined walls in the radiology department.

___

___

___

2. In what ways are X-rays utilized to diagnose illness?

___

___

___

3. In what ways are X-rays utilized to treat illness?

___

___

___

4. What is contrast media? How is it used and why?

____

____

____

____

____

5. To whom do X-ray films belong once they are taken and processed?

____

6. What special precautions should be taken when a patient is having excretory urography (IVP)?

____

____

____

Case Studies

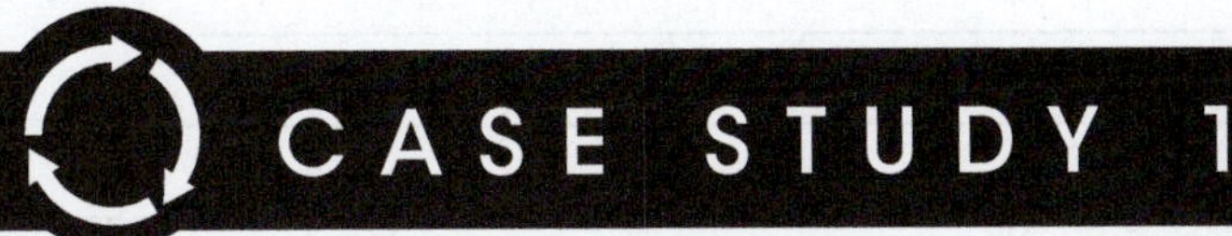

You begin working in a clinic where X-ray procedures are done. The provider has informed you that he will teach you the procedure for taking X-rays. In your state, special education and licensure are needed for a medical assistant to perform X-ray procedures. You also notice that no one in the clinic wears a dosimeter, although all are near the X-ray room during the day. Lead aprons are also not used on patients during X-ray procedures.

CASE STUDY REVIEW QUESTIONS

1. How will you handle this situation?

____

____

____

____

____

____

Research Activity

Using the search engine of your choice, discover how nuclear medicine is utilized to diagnose and treat disease. Prepare a PowerPoint presentation with a minimum of 5 slides to share with your class on your findings.

ATTRIBUTES OF PROFESSIONALISM

As a clinical medical assistant, how would you handle the situation if, in your state, taking X-rays is outside of your scope of practice? If you felt that you were outside of your comfort zone, and this type of examination is allowed in your state, how would you ask questions and communicate this to members of the health care team?

Name ______________________ Date __________ Score __________

CHAPTER 32

Rehabilitation and Therapeutic Modalities

VOCABULARY BUILDER

Misspelled Words

Find the words below that are misspelled; circle them, and correctly spell them in the spaces provided. Then write each correct vocabulary term next to the example below that best describes it.

activities of daily living	effleurage	modalities
ambulation	electromyography	range of motion
asistive device	gait belt	thermaltherapy
body mechanics	ghoniometer	ultrasound
contrackures	ghoniometry	vasalconstriction
criotherapy	hemaplegia	

______________ ______________ ______________

______________ ______________ ______________

______________ ______________ ______________

LEARNING REVIEW

1. ______________ When examining a new patient, a physical therapist must determine which of the physical agents, such as heat, cold, light, water, and electricity, will be most beneficial in treating the patient's condition.
2. ______________ Massage using circular motions with the palm of the hand that may ease muscle tissue.
3. ______________ As Margaret Thomas, diagnosed with Parkinson disease, began to experience balance problems and difficulties in walking, her physical therapist prescribed the use of high-frequency sound waves to generate heat in the deep tissue of her right leg, producing a therapeutic effect.

4. ________________________ Using extreme cold to destroy abnormal tissue is a treatment for abnormal cervical cells found with a Pap smear.

5. ________________________ Cold applications may be used to constrict blood vessels to slow or stop the flow of blood to an area.

6. ________________________ Lenny Taylor, suffering the early stages of dementia from Alzheimer disease, works with an occupational therapist to practice methods of making these everyday tasks easier to perform.

7. ________________________ Dr. Winston Lewis recommends this heat modality to help relieve Herb Fowler's chronic lower back pain, which is caused by strain on the back muscles created by the patient's overweight condition.

8. ________________________ When patient Linda Maier comes to Inner City Health Care describing a sore back and several recent falls, Dr. Osborne asks clinical medical assistant Joe Guerrero, CMA (AAMA), to secure a gait belt around Linda's waist and have her walk across the room. With Joe staying a step behind her and slightly to the side, Dr. Osborne carefully observes Linda's progress when performing this task.

9. ________________________ In order to diagnose carpal tunnel disorder, a recording of the electrical activity of muscle and nerve tissue is obtained.

10. ________________________ As a muscle atrophies, shrinking and losing its strength, joints become stiff and experience development of these deformities. Without constant exercise, the musculoskeletal system deteriorates.

11. ________________________ Dr. Angie Osborne recommends that patient Linda Maier begin to use a walker at home to prevent further falls. Joe Guerrero secures this item around Linda's waist and positions her inside the walker as he gives her verbal instructions to begin the procedure of learning to ambulate with a walker.

12. ________________________ Older adult patient Abigail Johnson is afraid that because she has diabetes mellitus she is at increased risk for stroke. "I don't want to end up a vegetable and a burden to my family," she tells Dr. Mark King, "all paralyzed on one side like that."

13. ________________________ Clinical medical assistant Joe Guerrero, CMA (AAMA), applies this practice of using certain key muscle groups together with correct body alignment to avoid injury when assisting patient Lenore McDonell in performing a transfer from her wheelchair to the examination table.

14. ________________________ Margaret Thomas's neurologist uses this instrument to measure the angle of her shoulder joint's ROM during a follow-up examination for Parkinson disease.

15. ________________________ Canes, walkers, and crutches are examples of walking aids.

16. ________________________ When lying flat with arms at the sides, the average person should be able to move from a 20-degree hyperextension of the elbow joint to a 150-degree flexion.

17. ________________________ A physical therapist uses the measurement of joint motion to help evaluate a patient's ROM.

Matching

Match each joint movement term listed below to its proper definition.

____ 1. Extension	A.	Moving the arm so the palm is up
____ 2. Circumduction	B.	Moving a body part outward
____ 3. Plantar flexion	C.	Straightening of a body part
____ 4. Dorsiflexion	D.	Motion toward the midline of the body
____ 5. Eversion	E.	Moving a body part inward
____ 6. Adduction	F.	Turning a body part around its axis
____ 7. Hyperextension	G.	A position of maximum extension, or extending a body part beyond its normal limits
____ 8. Flexion	H.	Motion away from the midline of the body
____ 9. Inversion	I.	Circular motion of a body part
____ 10. Pronation	J.	Moving the arm so the palm is down
____ 11. Supination	K.	Moving the foot downward at the ankle
____ 12. Rotation	L.	Moving the foot upward at the ankle joint
____ 13. Abduction	M.	Bending of a body part

LEARNING REVIEW

Short Answer

1. Name four types of exercise programs that are used for therapeutic or preventative purposes.

____

2. Using the four types of exercise programs identified in question 1 above, match each one to the example below that best describes it.

_______________ Pat Tidmarsh, who is suffering a sports injury to the muscles surrounding the knee, performs exercises with the help of a rubber exercise band.

_______________ Lourdes Austen performs self-directed exercises at home to improve the ROM and increase strength in her left arm, after lumpectomy and axillary lymph node dissection.

_______________ Lenore McDonell, who is confined to a wheelchair and unable to move her legs voluntarily, works regularly with a physical therapist to avoid atrophy and contractures in the legs and to improve overall circulation.

_______________ Luanne Moore, who is recovering from a shoulder injury, rebuilds upper body strength with a daily regimen of push-ups, first against the wall and then on the floor.

3. Therapeutic exercise is not the only way to treat painful joints or tissues. Many patients respond well to the therapeutic modalities of heat and cold, thermotherapy and cryotherapy. List six precautions that medical assistants must take when applying heat or cold modalities.

____

____

____

____

____

____

____

____

____

____

4. Identify each modality listed below as either a dry heat therapy (DHT), a moist heat therapy (MHT), a moist cold therapy (MCT), or a dry cold therapy (DCT) by placing the proper letters in the space provided. Then identify whether the modality can be performed at home by the patient, with or without caregiver assistance, or whether the modality must be performed in a clinical setting under the supervision of a health care professional.

_______ A. Ice pack ______________________

_______ B. Paraffin wax bath ______________________

_______ C. Cold compress ______________________

_______ D. Hot water bottle ______________________

_______ E. Warm compress ______________________

_______ F. Whirlpool bath ______________________

_______ G. Heating pad ______________________

_______ H. Warm soak of one extremity ______________________

_______ I. Warm pack ______________________

_______ J. Total body immersion in a Hubbard tank ______________________

5. For each of the following, identify the proper temperature and correct amount of time the modality should be administered to the patient. The first row has been completed for you as an example.

Modality	**Temperature**	**Time**
Aquamatic K-Pad for an older adult patient		
Paraffin wax bath for a patient with rheumatoid arthritis		
An ice pack for a patient with an ankle sprain		
Hot water bottle for an adult patient		
A warm compress to assist with drainage from a patient's skin infection		

Warm soak of the arm and hand for a patient with osteoarthritis

6. How do ultrasound waves best travel? What are the special concerns of ultrasound treatment, how long can ultrasound be administered, and who is authorized to perform ultrasound procedures on patients?

Image Labeling

Some patients require assistive devices to ambulate. Name each assistive device shown below, and then name the physical conditions for which each device is best suited to be used as part of a provider's treatment plan. The first row has been completed for you as an example.

	Name	**Uses**
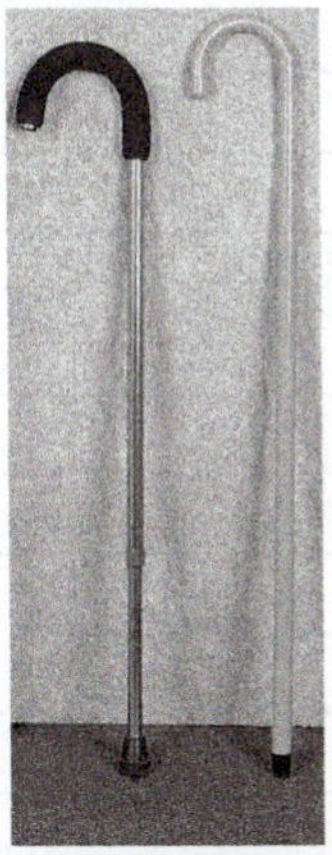		
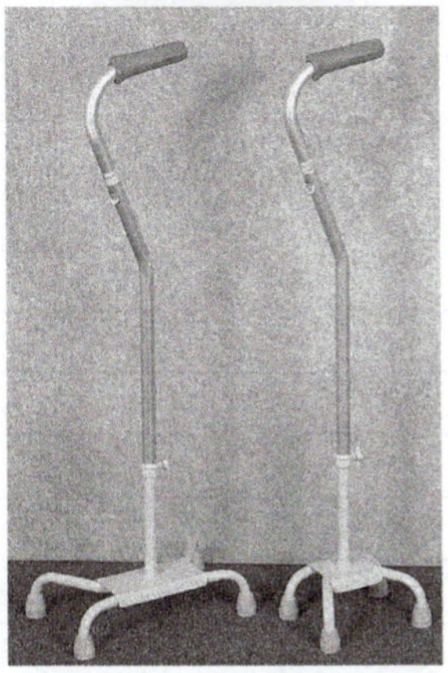		

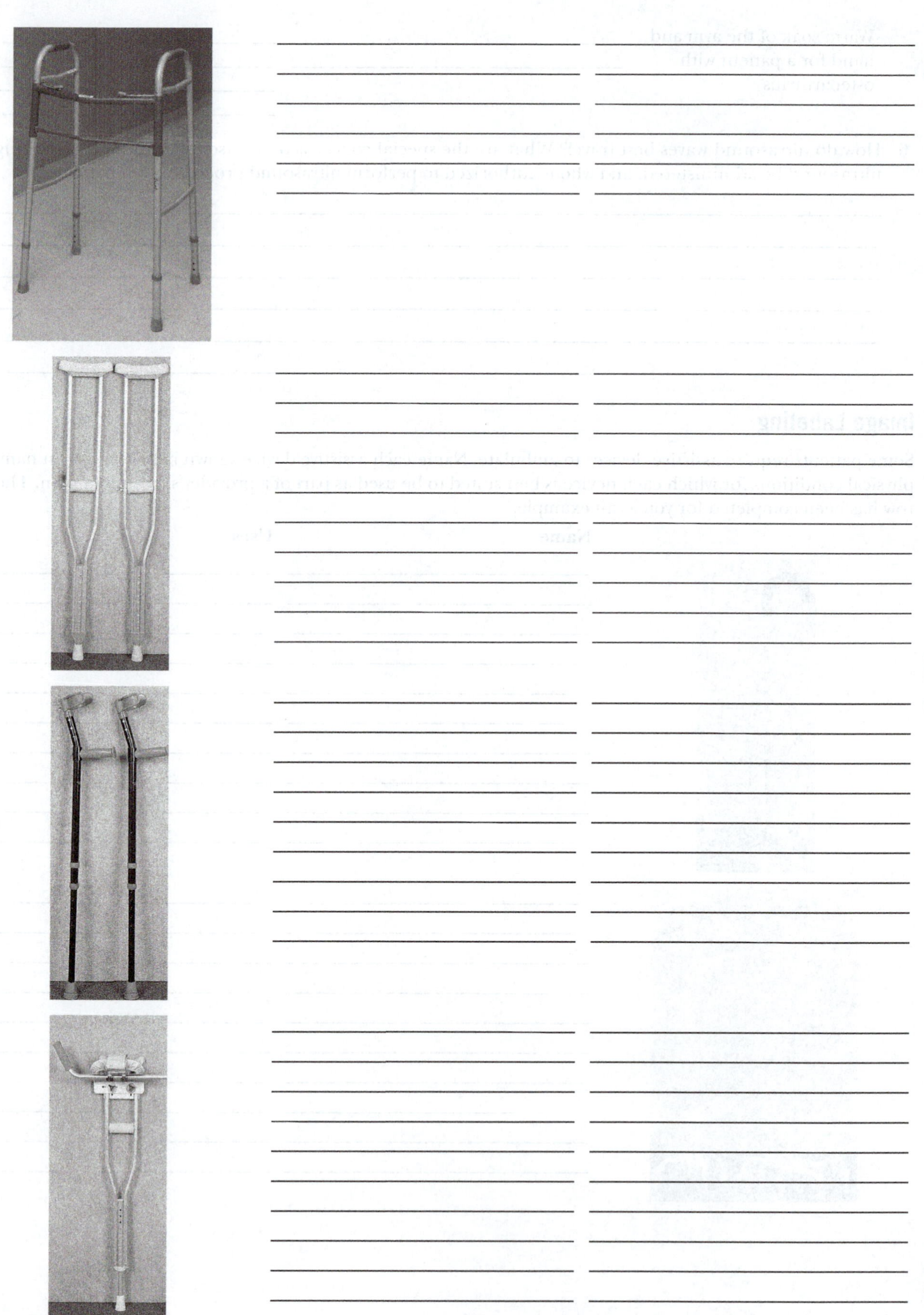

CERTIFICATION REVIEW

These questions are designed to mimic the certification examination. Select the best response.

1. The medical term for paralysis on one side is known as which of the following?
   a. Quadriplegia
   b. Paraplegia
   c. Hemiplegia
   d. Dysmenorrhea

2. Which of the following is a type of assistive device that does not require much upper body strength but is not recommended for older adults?
   a. Walker
   b. Cane
   c. Crutches
   d. Wheelchair
   e. Scooter

3. Which of the following are safety rules to be followed when moving a patient in a wheelchair?
   a. Always enter an elevator with the patient facing forward.
   b. Make sure the patient's feet are on the footrests prior to moving.
   c. Move down the center of corridors to avoid injuring the patient's elbows.
   d. Never bend your knees when assisting a patient to transfer.

4. Which of the following is the most effective type of crutch that may be used temporarily while a lower extremity heals?
   a. Axillary
   b. Forearm
   c. Platform
   d. Lofstrand
   e. Strutter

5. How many legs does a quad cane have?
   a. Two
   b. Four
   c. One
   d. Three

6. The use of activities to help restore independent functioning after an illness or injury is known as what?
   a. Physical therapy
   b. Rehabilitation medicine
   c. Speech therapy
   d. Sports medicine
   e. Play therapy

7. Which of the following is key when using lifting techniques?
   a. Use the large muscles of the legs and arms to lift
   b. Bend from the hips and knees, squat down, and push up with leg muscles
   c. Get as close as possible to the patient
   d. All of the above

8. The appropriate way to utilize a gait belt includes which activity?
   a. Lifting the patient by grasping the belt from underneath
   b. Lifting up
   c. Utilizing a firm grip on the patient's arms
   d. Bending at the waist and lifting the patient using your back muscles
   e. Both a and b

9. Walkers are used for patients who need which of the following?
   a. Maximum assistance
   b. Assistance with poor balance
   c. Stability
   d. All of the above

10. A patient with severe arthritis or poor use of their hands could utilize which of the following assistive devices?
   a. Axillary crutches
   b. Quad cane
   c. Platform crutches
   d. Rolling walker
   e. Strutter crutches

LEARNING APPLICATION

Critical Thinking

1. Define rehabilitation medicine and explain its importance in patient care.

2. Describe the procedure for measuring a patient for axillary crutches.

3. What kind of patient would need a forearm crutch?

4. In crutch-walking gaits, what is a *point*?

5. List the six safety rules for transporting a patient in a wheelchair.

6. What is joint range of motion, how is it measured, and how is the measurement expressed?

7. Describe how ultrasound works and identify the patient conditions for which it is an effective treatment.

8. Explain how to avoid internal damage to the patient when an ultrasound treatment is being performed.

Case Studies

CASE STUDY 1

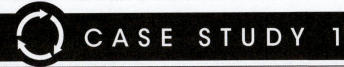

Ellen Armstrong, CMAS (AMT), performs the annual task of assembling and moving inactive patient files into a storage filing area for safekeeping. It is the end of the day and Ellen is tired and eager to finish the job—this task has never been one of Ellen's favorites. When she gets to filling the last of three cartons of files, Ellen moves the carton to a shelf, about shoulder height, in the storage room. She returns and decides to take both of the remaining cartons in one trip. Fatigued, she bends at the waist to pick them up.

CASE STUDY REVIEW QUESTION

1. Describe the proper lifting technique that Ellen should use.

CASE STUDY 2

After explaining the procedure to the patient Mary Craig and her son John, Gwen Carr, CMA (AAMA), applies a gait belt and begins the transfer of Mary from a car to a wheelchair in the parking lot of Inner City Health Care. Mary is an older adult who is blind, has diabetes mellitus, and is suffering from atrophy of the legs. Unfortunately, because of Mary's position in the car, she must be transferred with her weaker side closest to the wheelchair. The patient panics during the transfer and throws her arms around Gwen's neck as she is lifting and pivoting Mary to the right to position her in the wheelchair. The patient's son, John, rushes forward to grab onto his mother.

CASE STUDY REVIEW QUESTIONS

1. What is the best action of the medical assistant?

2. What is the best therapeutic response of the medical assistant?

3. Could the situation have been avoided? If so, how? If not, why not?

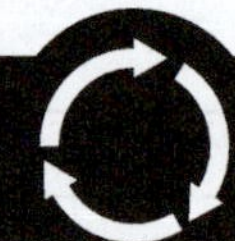

CASE STUDY 3

Dr. Ray Reynolds asks Thomas Myers, CCMA (NHA), to instruct patient Dottie Tate in the use of a walker to prevent further falls at home. Dottie is silent as Dr. Reynolds leaves the examination room and Thomas proceeds to set the walker correctly. However, when Dottie sees that Thomas must once again put her in a gait belt for her protection—the belt was used earlier in the examination to assess Dottie's ability to ambulate—the patient gets feisty. She is visibly tired and ready to go home. "I'll learn to use the walker if I have to, but I won't wear that infernal contraption. It makes me feel like a baby. And it's such a bother. Who wants to go through all that? We just don't need it."

CASE STUDY REVIEW QUESTIONS

1. What is the best action of the medical assistant?

2. What is the best therapeutic response of the medical assistant?

3. Could the situation have been avoided? If so, how? If not, why not?

Role-Play Activity

1. Assemble assistive devices:
   - Axillary crutches
   - Forearm crutches
   - Quad cane
   - Walker
   - Wheelchair

   Choose a partner from your classmates to play the part of the patient and instruct your "patient" on the use of various assistive devices. Change roles as medical assistant and patient.

2. With the same partner, use a gait belt to use correct body mechanics to safely transfer your patient from the examination table to a wheelchair. Switch roles and perform the activity again.

Research Activity

The World Health Organization has developed the International Classification of Functioning, Disability and Health, or ICF. ICF is a framework for addressing the more than a billion people worldwide with disabilities. Write a short definition paper exploring paradigm shifts in neurorehabilitation. Arrange to present the paper to your class.

ATTRIBUTES OF PROFESSIONALISM

1. What are some of the skills, talents, interests, and abilities a person would need to have to do well in rehabilitative medicine, taking into account the Attributes of Professionalism? List a dozen or more, and then consider and circle all of those that you possess. Which on the list could you learn in a rehabilitative medicine program (write an *S* for school), and which would be a natural part of your makeup (write an *N* for natural)? Is there a direct relation between the skills, talents, interests, and abilities you possess and those that you marked with an *N*? Discuss your results with a small group of fellow students. What conclusion(s) did you reach?

____

____

____

2. Much of rehabilitative medicine requires patient education on the various methodologies such as assistive devices, therapeutic modalities, and exercise. How would you be sure utilize the Attributes of Professionalism to attend to both the psychological and the physiologic aspects of the following conditions?
   a. Sally Roberts, age 25, is right-handed and has a right wrist fracture. Ms. Roberts lives alone with no family in the area. What type of postcasting instruction might be provided?

   ____

   ____

   ____

   b. Dylan McDaniel, age 85, has had a stroke and has left-sided weakness. He has recovered in the hospital and is now ready to be instructed regarding the use of a rolling walker. Mrs. McDaniel and their son, David, have accompanied him to this appointment. What type of instruction is appropriate for Mr. McDaniel?

   ____

   ____

   ____

Name ______________________________ Date ________ Score ________

CHAPTER **33**

Nutrition in Health and Disease

VOCABULARY BUILDER

Misspelled Words

Find the words below that are misspelled; circle them, and then correctly spell them in the spaces provided. Then fill in the blanks below with the correct vocabulary terms from the following list.

amino acids	digestion	nutrients
antioxident	electrolytes	nutrition
basal metabolic rate	extracellulare	oxydation
calories	fat-soluble	presearvatives
catalist	glycogen	processed foods
cellulose	homeostasis	saturated fats
coenzyeme	major mineral	trace minerals
diaretics	metabolism	water-soluable

________________ ________________ ________________

________________ ________________ ________________

________________ ________________ ________________

1. Artificial flavors, colors, and ________________ that keep food fresh longer are non-nutritive chemical substances commonly added to processed foods.
2. ________________ is the study of the intake of nutrients into the body and how the body processes and uses these nutrients.
3. Toxicity is most likely to occur with ________________ vitamins because they are stored in tissues composed of lipids and in the liver and are not carried easily into the bloodstream.
4. The best sources of complete proteins are meats and animal products such as milk and eggs; complete proteins contain all eight of the essential ________________.

5. Beverages that contain caffeine and alcohol, which are _______________, will cause the body to increase urinary output and lose water. These substances should be avoided when performing activities, such as a good physical workout, as well as when entering environments, such as an airplane passenger cabin, that promote dehydration.

6. A _______________ is a nonprotein substance that acts with a catalyst to facilitate chemical reactions in the body.

7. Chlorine (Cl) is a mineral with an important _______________ function, one that takes place outside the cells of body tissues in the spaces between layers or groups of cells.

8. The total of all changes, chemical and physical, that take place in the body is called _______________.

9. Some minerals are considered _______________ in that they become ionized and carry a positive or negative charge; these minerals must be carefully balanced in the body.

10. _______________ begins at the mouth with chewing and progresses through the gastrointestinal tract to the small intestine.

11. _______________ are ingested substances that help the body maintain a state of homeostasis.

12. The process of _______________ maintains a constant internal environment of the human body, including such functions as heartbeat, blood pressure, respiration, and body temperature.

13. A _______________ facilitates chemical reactions by speeding up the reaction time without the need for a high-energy output.

14. It is always important to analyze the nutritional labels on _______________ purchased in the supermarket.

15. Lard is one example of _______________, which have been found to increase the level of fats and cholesterol in the blood and are hydrogenated, or contain hydrogen.

16. The ability to reduce _______________ is a characteristic of vitamin E that has led some researchers to suggest that vitamin E may slow the aging process, although its true effectiveness has not yet been demonstrated.

17. The amount of energy a substance is able to supply is measured in _______________.

18. Potassium is one of the seven _______________ found in the body.

19. Vitamins that are _______________ must be constantly ingested to maintain proper blood levels, because these vitamins are not easily stored in the body.

20. Vitamin E is a fat-soluble vitamin that belongs to a group of compounds called _______________, which counteract the damaging effects of oxidation. Beta-carotene is another substance in this group.

21. Despite their name, _______________ are vital to body functioning and include molybdenum and fluorine.

22. Children, pregnant women, and people with a lean body mass will have a higher _______________ because it takes more energy to fuel the muscles than it does to store fat.

23. A type of carbohydrate, _______________, is derived from a plant source and supplies fiber in the human diet.

24. Ingested only in small quantities, _______________ is an important carbohydrate form for storage of glucose in the body.

LEARNING REVIEW

Short Answer

1. Vitamins are a class of nutrients in which each specific vitamin has a function entirely of its own. These complex molecules are required by the body in minute quantities. What are the two functions of vitamins in the body?

2. Identify the correct chemical name for each vitamin listed. Then describe what each vitamin does in the body to promote good health.

   A. One of the B-complex vitamins, also called nicotinic acid:

   B. Vitamin B_1:

   C. Vitamin E:

   D. Vitamin D:

   E. One of the B-complex vitamins, also called folacin:

   F. Vitamin A:

   G. Vitamin B_{12}:

   H. Vitamin C:

   I. Vitamin B_2:

   J. Vitamin B_6:

3. Nutrients are divided into two groups: those that provide energy and those that perform other essential roles to maintain the body. Identify the nutrients listed below as providing energy or providing maintenance by placing an *X* in the appropriate column.

	Energy	**Maintenance**
Vitamins		
Carbohydrates		
Fiber		
Minerals		
Lipids (fats)		
Proteins		
Water		

4. What three chemical elements do carbohydrates, fats, and proteins all contain?

____

____

5. Name the most important dietary complex carbohydrate. ______________________________

6. Name the only true essential fatty acid in the human diet. ______________________________

7. What chemical element does protein alone contain? ______________________________

8. What happens when the body does not have enough carbohydrates or fats in supply as an energy source? What effect does this have on the body?

____

____

9. Name two conditions associated with deficiencies in protein.

____

____

10. List two distinct ways in which minerals differ from vitamins.

____

____

____

11. For each food source, list the mineral or minerals that each provides.

A. Eggs: ______________________________

B. Milk: ______________________________

C. Cheese: ______________________________

D. Salmon: ______________________________

E. Bananas: ______________________________

F. Green vegetables: ______________________________

12. List six types of fiber that are carbohydrates.

____

____

13. What important fiber is *not* a carbohydrate?

14. Americans generally do not consume enough fiber. How much fiber should be consumed each day?

15. Why does brown rice contain more fiber than white rice?

16. What happens when the body takes in more calories than are expended by the body as energy?

17. What happens when the body uses more energy than the calories it takes in?

18. What is the ideal percentage of total calories for adults that should be consumed as carbohydrates, fats, and proteins?

19. Compare the advantages and disadvantages of the following diets: U.S. Southern, Jewish, and Japanese.

20. Obesity is a major health concern in the United States and often begins in childhood. What can you do as a medical assistant to aid parents to help their children avoid obesity?

Matching

Review the substances listed in Column A. In Column B, identify whether each substance is a water-soluble vitamin (WSV), fat-soluble vitamin (FSV), major mineral (MM), or trace mineral (TM). Then, match each description in Column C to the appropriate substance in Column A, using the blank spaces at the beginning of each example to enter your answers. The first item has been completed for you as a guide.

	Column A	Column B	Column C
______	1. Sulfur	__________	A. This substance works with potassium to maintain proper water balance and proper pH balance; the two also are involved in muscular nerve conduction and excitability.
______	2. Vitamin B_{12}	__________	B. This substance is part of the pigment rhodopsin found in the eye and is responsible in part for vision, especially night vision.
______	3. Iron	__________	C. This substance is vital to life because of its role in the heme molecule, which carries oxygen to every cell in the body.
______	4. Vitamin K	__________	D. Rickets and osteomalacia are diseases caused by deficiencies in this substance; when deficiencies occur, usually in childhood, malformation of the skeleton is seen.
______	5. Sodium	__________	E. This member of the B-complex, together with pantothenic acid, is generally responsible for energy metabolism.
______	6. Pyridoxine	__________	F. Because this substance is found only in foods from animal sources, such as liver, kidney, and dairy products, pernicious anemia, the result of deficiencies, may be a problem for some vegetarians.
______	7. Iodine	__________	G. This substance, found in rice, beans, and yeast, is important in protein metabolism.
______	8. Biotin	__________	H. This substance is a component of one of the amino acids and is found in protein; it is also involved in energy metabolism.
______	9. Retinol	__________	I. About half of the body's requirement for this substance is fulfilled through synthesis by intestinal bacteria; bile is required for its absorption into the bloodstream.
______	10. Vitamin D	__________	J. This substance is found only in the thyroid hormones; without it, the thyroid gland would be unable to regulate the overall metabolism of the body.

CERTIFICATION REVIEW

These questions are designed to mimic the certification examination. Select the best response.

1. Carbohydrates, fats, and proteins have one thing in common. What is it?
   a. High calcium content
   b. Ability to convert into energy
   c. Low sodium content
   d. All of the above

2. Which of the following is an example of a monosaccharide?
   a. Fructose
   b. Sucrose
   c. Glucose
   d. Amylose
   e. Both a and c

3. What is the name for the compounds composed of carbon, hydrogen, and oxygen that exist as triglycerides in the body?
   a. Fats
   b. Fiber
   c. Vitamins
   d. Minerals

4. Which of the following is the basic structural unit of a protein?
   a. Simple sugar
   b. Complex sugar
   c. Lipids
   d. Starch
   e. Amino acids

5. Each gram of a carbohydrate contains how many calories?
   a. Four
   b. Eight
   c. Ten
   d. Twelve

6. Chemical digestion begins with amylase that is secreted by which of the following body structures?
   a. Lining of the stomach
   b. Pancreas
   c. Salivary glands
   d. Small intestine
   e. Tongue

7. The body stores glucose in which of the following forms?
   a. Insulin
   b. Glycogen
   c. Fat
   d. Bone

8. Xerophthalmia is a deficiency of which of the following vitamins?
   a. Vitamin A
   b. Vitamin B
   c. Vitamin C
   d. Vitamin D
   e. Vitamin E

9. Pyridoxine is the name of which vitamin?
   a. Vitamin A
   b. Vitamin B_{12}
   c. Vitamin B_6
   d. Vitamin C

10. During which of the following body processes are free radicals produced?
    a. When amino acids are broken down
    b. When the body uses oxygen to burn food for energy
    c. When the body fails to excrete nitrogen
    d. When DNA breaks down
    e. When vitamins are absorbed

LEARNING APPLICATION

Critical Thinking

1. Identify each organ of the digestive system below. Describe the healthy functioning of each organ in the space provided. Then, using a medical dictionary or encyclopedia, look up each organ and list one common disorder that would adversely affect the digestive process.

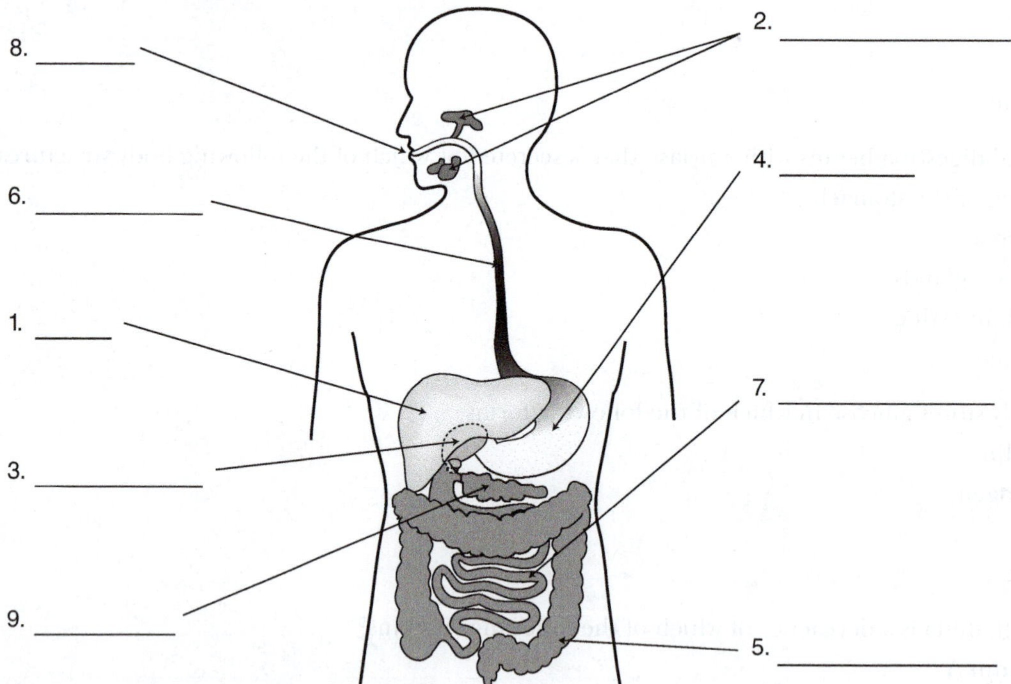

Healthy Function	**Common Disorders**
1. ______________________	______________________
2. ______________________	______________________
3. ______________________	______________________
4. ______________________	______________________
5. ______________________	______________________
6. ______________________	______________________
7. ______________________	______________________
8. ______________________	______________________
9. ______________________	______________________

2. When helping patients modify their diets, medical assistants need to be knowledgeable about the nutrients in the food we eat. The nutritional analysis label on the back or side of a food package is helpful when figuring out the levels of fat, cholesterol, sodium, carbohydrates, protein, and vitamins contained in a particular food. Obtain a food label and answer the following questions.

   A. The percentage of daily values listed on a food label report the amount of a nutrient obtained by eating how many servings of a product? _____

   B. The percentages are based on a _____-calorie diet.

   C. The listing for total carbohydrates is broken down into what two additional listings? Which type of carbohydrate is more beneficial and why?

   ____

   ____

   D. Why is a high-fiber diet important?

   ____

   ____

   ____

3. Compare the nutrition label from a box of muesli with fruit, nuts, and seeds with the label from a package of pretzel snacks. Which is more nutritious and why? Note that one serving of the muesli, a half cup or 55 grams, is roughly equivalent to 2 servings of pretzels, 14 pretzels or 60 grams.

____

____

____

____

____

____

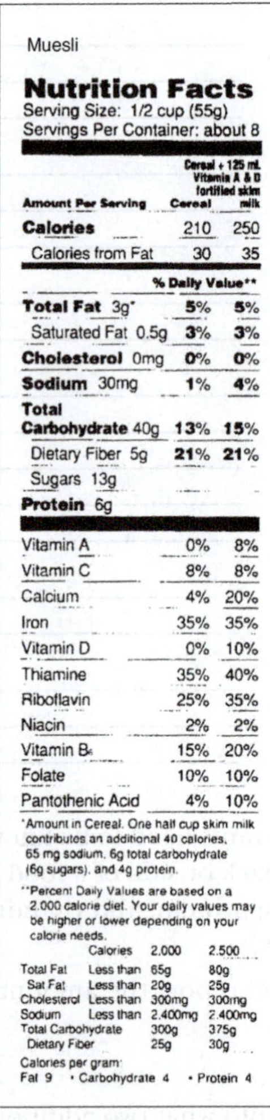

Muesli

Nutrition Facts

Serving Size: 1/2 cup (55g)
Servings Per Container: about 8

Amount Per Serving	Cereal	Cereal + 125 mL Vitamin A & D fortified skim milk
Calories	210	250
Calories from Fat	30	35
	% Daily Value**	
Total Fat 3g*	**5%**	**5%**
Saturated Fat 0.5g	**3%**	**3%**
Cholesterol 0mg	**0%**	**0%**
Sodium 30mg	**1%**	**4%**
Total Carbohydrate 40g	**13%**	**15%**
Dietary Fiber 5g	**21%**	**21%**
Sugars 13g		
Protein 6g		
Vitamin A	0%	8%
Vitamin C	8%	8%
Calcium	4%	20%
Iron	35%	35%
Vitamin D	0%	10%
Thiamine	35%	40%
Riboflavin	25%	35%
Niacin	2%	2%
Vitamin B_6	15%	20%
Folate	10%	10%
Pantothenic Acid	4%	10%

*Amount in Cereal. One half cup skim milk contributes an additional 40 calories, 65 mg sodium, 6g total carbohydrate (6g sugars), and 4g protein.

**Percent Daily Values are based on a 2,000 calorie diet. Your daily values may be higher or lower depending on your calorie needs.

	Calories	2,000	2,500
Total Fat	Less than	65g	80g
Sat Fat	Less than	20g	25g
Cholesterol	Less than	300mg	300mg
Sodium	Less than	2,400mg	2,400mg
Total Carbohydrate		300g	375g
Dietary Fiber		25g	30g

Calories per gram:
Fat 9 • Carbohydrate 4 • Protein 4

Pretzels

Nutrition Facts

Serving Size: 7 Pretzels (30g)
Servings Per Container: 9.4

Amount Per Serving	
Calories 120	Calories from Fat 10
	% Daily Value*
Total Fat 1g	**2%**
Saturated Fat 0g	**0%**
Cholesterol 0g	**0%**
Sodium 360mg	**15%**
Total Carbohydrate 24g	**8%**
Dietary Fiber 1g	**4%**
Sugars 1g	
Protein 3g	

Vitamin A 0% ∑ Vitamin C 0%
Calcium 0% ∑ Iron 2%

*Percent Daily Values are based on a 2,000 calorie diet. Your daily values may be higher or lower depending on your calorie needs:

		Calories 2,000	2,500
Total Fat	Less than	65g	80g
Sat Fat	Less than	20g	25g
Cholesterol	Less than	300mg	300mg
Sodium	Less than	2,400mg	2,400mg
Total Carbohydrate		300g	375g
Dietary Fiber		25g	30g

Calories per gram:
Fat 9 ∑ Carbohydrate 4 ∑ Protein 4

Ingredients: Unbleached Wheat Flour, Water, Corn Syrup, Partially Hydrogenated Vegetable Oil (Soybean), Yeast Salt, Bicarbonates and Carbonates of Sodium.

4. Evaluate your own diet. Write down every item you eat in a day and find the values of the nutrients contained in the foods. A medical dictionary is a good source for listing the nutrient value of selected foods. If you are eating prepared foods, read the package food label. Remember, you are trying to get an idea of your average daily diet, so do not change your diet for your analysis unless you plan to maintain it. What is the balance of your energy nutrients? Are you getting enough vitamins and minerals? Are you getting adequate fiber? What modifications could you make?

____

____

____

____

5. Write a response to a teenage girl who refuses to gain weight during her pregnancy.

____

____

____

____

____

____

____

Case Studies

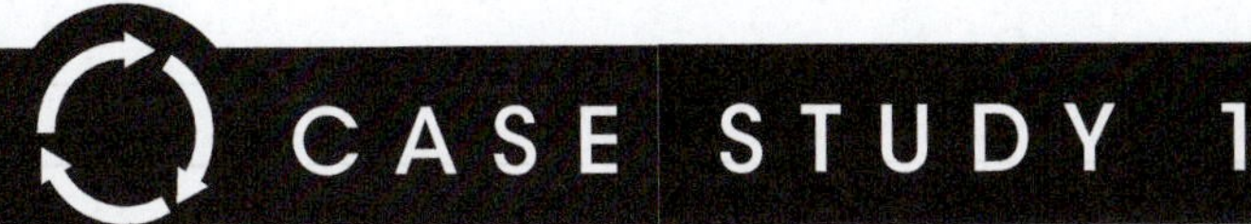

Dr. Mark King has confirmed that patient Mary O'Keefe is pregnant with her third child.

CASE STUDY REVIEW QUESTIONS

1. Name two minerals that Mary must increase the intake of in her diet.

____

2. Name three reasons a woman needs to increase her intake of nutrients and calories when she is pregnant.

____

____

____

____

3. What dietary supplements usually need to be added to a baby's diet?

____

CASE STUDY 2

Lourdes Austen, a breast cancer survivor, regularly attends a support group for breast patients with cancer and survivors held once a month. Lourdes finds the group a great source of encouragement, information, and support—a safe place to discuss her feelings and concerns about breast cancer. The group is planning a session to talk about nutrition issues, and Lourdes asks clinical medical assistant Nancy McFarland, RMA (AMT), if she would like to attend the meeting with her to contribute to the group's discussion. With permission from clinic manager Marilyn Johnson and Lourdes's provider Dr. Mark King, Nancy attends the meeting. The group members are enthusiastic and ask Nancy many questions, including the following: Why is good nutrition important for patients with cancer? I don't have much appetite anymore and get nauseous all the time. What can I do? I keep hearing about those macrobiotic diets. Are they any good? Should I try them?

CASE STUDY REVIEW QUESTIONS

1. What information can Nancy give in answer to the question regarding the importance of good nutrition for patients with cancer?

2. What suggestion can Nancy offer to patients who have no appetite and have nausea or vomiting?

3. What can Nancy tell the group about macrobiotic diets?

4. What is the role of the medical assistant in attending the breast cancer support group meeting?

Calorie Calculating Activity

1. An 8-fluid-ounce serving of 1% fat soy milk contains 110 calories with 2 grams of total fat, 20 grams of total carbohydrates, and 4 grams of total protein. Calculate the total number of calories from each energy nutrient (show your calculations in the space provided below).
   Number of calories from fat: __
   Number of calories from carbohydrates: __
   Number of calories from protein: __

2. Now calculate the percentage of total calories from each energy nutrient.
   Percentage of calories from fat: __
   Percentage of calories from carbohydrates: __
   Percentage of calories from protein: ____

3. Compare the percentages of total calories due to fat, carbohydrates, and protein found in soy milk with the percentages you calculated for one serving of peanut butter in the textbook's Critical Thinking box on page 1041. How do the percentages relate to the ideal percentages for optimum energy balance in the body?

____

____

____

____

Research Activity

In 2011, the USDA changed the Food Guide Pyramid to MyPlate as a guide to recommended nutritional intake for Americans. What are the significant changes that occurred with this shift? How are these recommendations formulated? Write a short description of these changes, make a prediction for future change recommendations, and present them to your class.

ATTRIBUTES OF PROFESSIONALISM

Bai Wang, a 48-year-old Chinese American patient of Dr. Reynolds, is newly diagnosed with type 2 diabetes. Dr. Reynolds has asked you to initiate dietary education. What cultural considerations must be taken into account prior to initiating your teaching session? Utilizing the Attributes of Professionalism, how would you discover these important cultural keys to success for Mr. Wang?

____

____

____

____

____

____

____

____

____

____

____

____

Name ______________________ Date ________ Score ________

CHAPTER 34

Basic Pharmacology

VOCABULARY BUILDER

Misspelled Words

Find the words in Column A that are misspelled; circle them, and then correctly spell them in the spaces provided. Then match each vocabulary term below with the correct definition in Column B.

	Column A	Correct Spelling	Column B
____	1. Abuse	____________	A. Term used to describe when a licensed practitioner gives an order that is transmitted to a pharmacy to be filled
____	2. Transdermal	____________	B. A biological macromolecule or cellular component used as a pharmaceutical
____	3. Absorption	____________	C. A term in pharmacokinetics that refers to assessing the expected in vivo biological equivalence of two proprietary preparations of a drug
____	4. Pruritis	____________	D. An allergic hypersensitivity reaction of the body to a foreign protein or drug
____	5. Administer	____________	E. A drug whose manufacture, possession, and use is regulated by the government
____	6. Bioequavalent	____________	F. A system of medication delivery that includes a patch with a concentration of medication absorbed through the skin
____	7. Controlled substance	____________	G. To give medication to patient to be used at another time
____	8. Anaphalaxis	____________	H. The process by which a drug is excreted from the body
____	9. Biopharmaceutical	____________	I. The study of drugs; the science dealing with their history, origin, sources, physical and chemical properties, uses, and effects on living organisms

_____ 10. Contradictation _______________ J. The study of the response to medications based on one's genetic inheritance

_____ 11. Farmacology _______________ K. The chemical alteration that a drug undergoes in the body, usually in the liver

_____ 12. Distribution _______________ L. Medications derived from animals

_____ 13. Biotransphormation _______________ M. To give a medication to a patient by mouth, injection, or any other method of delivery

_____ 14. Perscribe _______________ N. Any symptom or circumstance for which an otherwise approved form of treatment is inadvisable

_____ 15. Uriticaria _______________ O. The medical term for severe itching of the skin

_____ 16. Dispense _______________ P. The process by which a drug passes into the body fluids or tissues

_____ 17. Pharmazooticals _______________ Q. The medical term for hives

_____ 18. Pharmacogenomics _______________ R. The misuse of legal and illegal drugs

_____ 19. Elimination _______________ S. The process by which a drug is transported from the blood to the intended site of action

LEARNING REVIEW

Short answer

1. Under federal law, providers who prescribe, administer, or dispense controlled substances must register with the DEA and renew their registration as required by state law. Describe the five schedules of classification for controlled substances and give an example for each.

____

____

____

____

____

____

____

____

2. For each of the following, identify whether the drug involved is an OTC medication (OTC) or a prescribed medication (PM). What patient guidelines for proper use are illustrated in each example?

_______ A. Nora Fowler insists that Dr. Winston Lewis cannot help her rheumatoid arthritis and that simple ibuprofen is all she needs. Nora buys bulk generic bottles of ibuprofen at the drugstore for her rheumatoid arthritis and takes as many as she needs to help ease the painful inflammation in her joints and tissues.

_______ B. When Jim Marshall experiences extreme stress while finishing the architectural designs for a new office building in the community, his girlfriend offers him a tablet or two of lorazepam, a benzodiazepine drug used to treat anxiety and insomnia. "Here, Dr. King gave me these, and they work great," she says. "You can't drive when you take this stuff, though. Oh, and these pills are about 2 years old, but I'm sure they'll still work fine."

_______ C. At the slightest sniffle or sneeze, Lenore McDonell takes the strongest multisymptom cold medication she can find. Her philosophy is: "I might as well knock it out of my system."

_______ D. Abigail Johnson hates taking so many medications. So every now and then, when she feels especially good, Abigail just decides to stop taking the antihypertensive drug that is part of Dr. Mark King's treatment plan to control Abigail's high blood pressure. On a bad day, she'll take an extra pill.

_______ E. Patty McLean is susceptible to recurrent colds and ear infections. Patty's symptoms are hard to control because she will almost always stop taking the antibiotics when she starts to feel better and she does not finish the entire regimen recommended by Dr. Lewis.

3. Proper disposal of drugs has become increasingly important. How should outdated medications be disposed of?

4. The most frequently used routes of administering medication are oral and parenteral. List seven additional routes of administration.

____

____

____

5. Name two more recently developed systems of drug delivery. Describe each and note their specific advantages.

____

____

____

____

____

6. List four examples of the ways in which drugs may be classified, or arranged, in groups.

____

____

____

____

7. For each drug action, identify the correct drug classification. Then list one example of a drug contained in each class. The first row has been completed as an example for you.

Action	Classification	Drug Example
Controls or stops bleeding		
Prevents or relieves nausea and vomiting		
Neutralizes acid		
Decreases blood pressure		
Reduces fever		
Loosens and promotes normal bowel elimination		
Prevents conception		
Kills or destroys malignant cells		
Prevents or relieves diarrhea		
Produces a calming effect without causing sleep		

CERTIFICATION REVIEW

These questions are designed to mimic the certification examination. Select the best response.

1. What is true about over-the-counter drugs?
   a. They require a prescription.
   b. They are safe to use without the provider's supervision.
   c. They can be taken in unlimited quantities.
   d. None of the above.

2. Federal law requires that at the end of the workday, controlled substances that are used on the clinic premises must be managed in which of the following ways?
   a. Locked in a provider's office by a provider
   b. Counted, verified by two individuals, and recorded on an audit sheet
   c. Discarded by flushing down the toilet or hopper
   d. Returned to a pharmacy
   e. Held until a local pharmacy's "take-back" day

3. An inventory record of Schedule II drugs must be submitted to the Drug Enforcement Administration (DEA) how often?
   a. Weekly
   b. Monthly
   c. Yearly
   d. Every 2 years

4. The *Physician's Desk Reference* contains which of the following information?
   a. Brand and generic names of medications
   b. Classification or category of medications
   c. Product information
   d. Methods of administration
   e. All of the above

5. Which of the following is an example of an OTC drug?
   a. Analgesic ibuprofen
   b. Vasodilator nitroglycerin
   c. Antitussive codeine
   d. Narcotic morphine

6. What is the term for when a drug acts on the area to which it is administered?
   a. Systemic action
   b. Remote action
   c. Local action
   d. Conductive action
   e. None of the above

7. The four principal factors that affect drug action are absorption, distribution, biotransformation, and which of the following?
   a. Elimination
   b. Interaction
   c. Contraindication
   d. Excretion

8. By law, outdated and expired controlled substances must be handled in which of the following ways?
   a. Handed over to your local law enforcement agency
   b. Thrown away in the trash
   c. Returned to a pharmacy on a designated "take-back" day
   d. Flushed down a toilet
   e. Donated to the local veterinarian for animal use

9. What are the most frequently used routes of administering medication?
   a. Inhalation and sublingual
   b. Parenteral and inhalation
   c. Oral and parenteral
   d. Transdermal and oral

10. Which of the following is a controlled substance–related responsibility of the medical assistant?
    a. Provide security for prescription pads
    b. Properly dispose of and document the disposal of expired drugs
    c. Maintain legal inventories of medications
    d. Participate in an end-of-shift narcotic count
    e. All of these

LEARNING APPLICATION

Critical Thinking

1. What factor related to determining the route selection for administering a medication is illustrated by each example below, and why?

   A. A patient diagnosed with insulin-dependent diabetes mellitus performs three self-injections of insulin daily, according to the provider's treatment plan.

   ____

   ____

   ____

   B. Chemotherapeutic drugs are used to attack cancer cells wherever they may occur in a patient's body, and usually they are administered intravenously.

   ____

   ____

   ____

C. A patient in a nursing home who is in the end stages of Parkinson disease is bedridden, has trouble swallowing, and suffers from dementia. The patient, who is also suffering from angina as a result of poor blood circulation, is prescribed a nitroglycerin transdermal system instead of a sublingual dosage, to be held under the tongue, or time-released capsule to swallow.

____

____

____

____

Case Studies

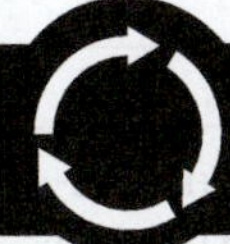

CASE STUDY 1

While Nancy McFarland, RMA (AMT), a clinical medical assistant at Inner City Health Care is performing her shift duties, she notices a fellow employee exhibiting strange behavior. Gwen Carr, CMA (AAMA), is usually the model of efficiency. Nancy has always known Gwen to be alert, friendly, and able to handle difficult clinical situations with grace under pressure. Lately, however, when Nancy asks Gwen questions, Gwen seems irritable and easily confused. Nancy also notices Gwen exhibiting a sloppy technique during routine clinical procedures. Nancy is disturbed by Gwen's erratic behavior but does not mention anything to anyone because they are friends. But while counting the contents of the controlled substance cabinet in preparation for the end of her shift, Nancy notices that a bottle of phenobarbital is missing. Nancy knows that clinic manager Marilyn Johnson will arrive shortly to verify and record the inventory count. Nancy is now worried that perhaps Gwen is to blame for the missing drugs but is afraid of jumping to conclusions and of angering Gwen. Nancy knows Gwen is in the staff lounge preparing to leave for a dinner break.

CASE STUDY REVIEW QUESTIONS

1. What is Nancy's first action under the circumstances? Should she confront Gwen?

____

____

____

____

____

2. What special responsibilities do health care professionals, including medical assistants, have regarding the misuse or abuse of legal and illegal drugs?

____

____

____

____

____

____

____

Research Activities

The PDR is an invaluable resource and one of the most widely used publications in the medical industry. The annually updated publication is usually available in most clinics and medical offices. It provides medical professionals with practical information about thousands of medications and includes other useful data, such as lists of drugs new to the market and those that have been discontinued. It is essential that medical assistants become familiar with the publication and learn how to access the wealth of information stored within.

1. Use the PDR to locate the pertinent information for each of the following scenarios. Then identify the drug's source or method of production.

   A. Herb Fowler, Dr. Winston Lewis's patient, calls to report he is experiencing nausea, a symptom he believes may be a negative reaction to the Chronulac Syrup Dr. Lewis recently prescribed for Herb's chronic constipation. Using the PDR, locate the following information:

   Chronulac Syrup's generic name: ___

   The sugar that Chronulac Syrup contains is ___

   Identify the drug's source or method of production:

   B. Another patient of Dr. Lewis's, Michael Zamboni, has recently been diagnosed with insulin-dependent type II diabetes. Dr. Lewis prescribes Humulin. Using the PDR, find the following information:

   Humulin's generic name: ___

   Identify the drug's source or method of production: ___

   C. Susan Marshall, a new patient of Dr. Mark King, acquired a high-pressure job about a month ago. Recently, she has been reporting an upset stomach, which has been attributed to her stressful job and poor eating habits. Dr. King orders prescription-strength Pepcid for Susan. Using the PDR, locate the following information:

   Pepcid's generic name: ___

   Pepcid's active ingredient: ___

   Identify the drug's source or method of production: ___

2. Camille Saunders, another patient of Dr. King, has been taking Ortho Tri-Cyclen, an oral contraceptive, for 6 months. It has just been discovered that Camille has epilepsy. Using the PDR, locate the following information:

   A. Does Ortho Tri-Cyclen have any known contraindications to any drugs used in the treatment of epilepsy, and if so, which drugs? ___

   B. Identify the drug's source or method of production. ___

ATTRIBUTES OF PROFESSIONALISM

1. Choose a partner from your class or practice with a member of your family. Either create a fictional list of medications or with a list of your family member's medication, create medicine cards to be carried with them at all times. On the card, list the drug, strength, and dose. Speaking at the level of the "patient's" understanding, explain the reason for taking the medication, the most appropriate dosing schedule, side effects, and other important aspects of each particular medication.

2. Research the guidelines for your state with regard to a medical assistant's role in the refill of medications. Create three scenarios where refilling a medication falls within your scope of practice in your state. If some refills lie outside of your scope of practice, how would you communicate this to your health care team members?

____

____

____

____

Name ______________________ Date ________ Score ________

CHAPTER 35

Calculation of Medication Dosage and Medication Administration

VOCABULARY BUILDER

Misspelled Words

Find the words below that are misspelled; circle them, and correctly spell them in the spaces provided. Then fill in each blank in the sentences below with the correct vocabulary term.

administering	hypoxemia	port
apnea	meniskis	precipitate
body surface area	namogram	retrolental fibroplasia
compounding	parentral	status asthmaticus
dispensing	pharmakokinetics	unit dose

______________________ ______________________ ______________________

______________________ ______________________ ______________________

1. The absence of breathing is termed ____________________.
2. ____________________ describes asthma attacks that occur in rapid succession or a sustained attack that does not respond to usual intervention.
3. ____________________ is a highly accurate method for calculating medication dosages for infants and children up to 12 years of age.
4. The study of the movement of drugs within the body is referred to as ____________________.
5. A lack of oxygen in the blood is ____________________.
6. The convex or concave upper surface of a column of liquid in a container is known as the ____________________.

7. Large-vein access that is surgically created and used for long-term use as with chemotherapy is called a ____________________.

8. A ____________________ is a graph that shows the relationship among numerical values.

9. ____________________ is a disease of the eye that is related to premature birth and the administration of oxygen therapy.

10. The term ____________________ describes a route other than the alimentary canal for injection of a liquid substance into the body.

11. Federal and state codes exist regarding administering and ____________________ medications and there is variation between the two. Medications that are prepared for specific people based on a carefully written prescription are formulated in a ____________________ pharmacy.

12. ____________________ is a substance in the form of fine particles that separates from a solution that is allowed to stand for a period of time.

13. A ____________________ is a premeasured amount of medication, individually packaged on a per dose basis.

14. Caution must be utilized when ____________________ the first dose of a medication to a patient.

LEARNING REVIEW

Short Answer

1. Identify the following measures as weight (W) or volume (V). Then name the measure each abbreviation stands for and what system of measurement it belongs to. The first row has been completed as an example for you.

Weight	Volume	Abbreviation	Measure	System
		g/Gm	Gram	Metric
		tbsp	________	________
		mL	________	________
		qt	________	________
		gtt	________	________
		µg	________	________

2. Perform the following conversions:

a. 4 tsp = ____ mL

b. 7 kg = ____ lb

c. 3.5 in. = ____ cm

d. 1,200 mg = ____ g

e. 8 mL = ____ gtt

3. What are proportions? How are proportions useful in calculating dosages of medication?

____

____

____

____

____

4. Identify the type of syringe typically used for each of the following. List the size and calibration as well.

Purpose	**Type**	**Size**	**Calibration**
Venipuncture	____________	______	__________________
Insulin administration	____________	______	__________________
Allergy testing	____________	______	__________________

5. For each syringe–needle combination below, identify the most likely parenteral route: subcutaneous injection (SC), intramuscular injection (IM), or intradermal injection (ID). Also identify the proper angle of injection.

	Route	**Angle of Injection**
3-mL syringe/22-G, 1½-inch needle	_____	__________________
1-mL syringe/25-G, ¾-inch needle	_____	__________________
U-100 (1 mL)/26-G, ½-inch needle	_____	__________________
3-mL syringe/25-G, ¾-inch needle	_____	__________________

CERTIFICATION REVIEW

These questions are designed to mimic the certification examination. Select the best response.

1. The hard copy of a prescription is filed and kept for a minimum of how many years?
   a. 10
   b. 7
   c. 5
   d. Indefinitely

2. What is the term that describes the portion of the prescription that gives directions to the patient?
   a. Superscription
   b. Inscription
   c. Subscription
   d. Signature
   e. Description

3. Injections should be avoided in which areas?
   a. Burns
   b. Inflamed areas
   c. Previous injection sites
   d. All of the above

4. Dosage of insulin is always measured in which of the following?
   a. Cubic centimeters
   b. Milliliters
   c. Units
   d. Milliequivalents
   e. Microliters

5. Which of the following terms describes the hollow core of a needle?
   a. Bevel
   b. Gauge
   c. Lumen
   d. Hilt

6. What is a potential hazard of medication administration by intramuscular injection?
   a. Injury to bone
   b. Breaking of the needle
   c. Injecting into a blood vessel
   d. Injury to a nerve
   e. All of the above

7. The gentle pulling back on the plunger of the syringe to ensure the needle tip is not in a blood vessel is termed which of the following?
   a. Injection
   b. Aspiration
   c. Instillation
   d. Infusion

8. A disposable plastic tube that has small holes to be inserted in the nares is referred to as which of the following?
   a. Mask
   b. Nasal cannula
   c. Nasal catheter
   d. Trach
   e. Positive pressure

9. Medications that are irritating to the tissues should be injected using what method?
   a. Intramuscular
   b. Slow
   c. Z-track
   d. Subcutaneous

10. Rapid response to a medication can be expected with which method of administration?
    a. Oral
    b. Intravenous
    c. Intramuscular
    d. Transdermal
    e. Both b and c

LEARNING APPLICATION

Critical Thinking

1. Describe the process to follow to determine a particular state's law regarding a medical assistant administering medications.

2. What is a medication order? Describe its purpose.

3. Name and describe factors that can affect medication dosage. Explain why and how the dosage is affected.

4. Name two methods used to calculate pediatric dosages of medication.

5. List and describe the "Six Rights" of medication administration.

6. A fellow student tells you that she accidentally gave a patient the incorrect dose of medication. Explain in detail what should be done.

7. You accidentally stick yourself with a contaminated needle. What are the correct steps to take?

Calculation Challenges

1. Calculate the following dosages according to body surface area (BSA):
   a. If the adult dose of EES tabs is 400 mg every 6 hours, what is the dosage for a child who is 35 inches tall and weighs 28 pounds (BSA 0.57)?

   b. If the adult dose of penicillin V potassium, USP, is 250 mg every 6 to 8 hours, what is the dosage for a child who is 24 inches tall and weighs 35 pounds (BSA 0.56)?

2. Calculate the following dosages according to kilogram of body weight:
   a. The provider orders Augmentin 20 mg/kg/day for Sally Whitney, who weighs 72 pounds. The dose is to be divided and given every 8 hours. What is the total dose? What is the dose to be given every 8 hours?

   ____

   b. The provider orders Cefadyl 40 mg/kg for George Kipperley, who weighs 78 pounds. The dosage is to be divided into four equal doses. What is the total dosage? What is the amount to be given in four equal doses?

   ____

3. The provider orders 125 mg Diamox for an adult patient. On hand you have 250 mg tablets. How many tablets will you give to your patient?

   ____

4. The provider orders 250 mg of Tagamet liquid. On hand you have 300 mg/5 mL. How many milliliters will you give?

   ____

Case Studies

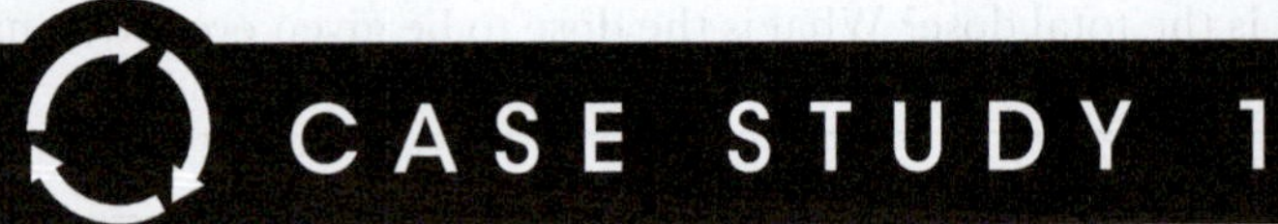

Louise Kipperley comes to Inner City Urgent Care when she experiences her third severe migraine headache this month. The headache has lasted 2 days, and Louise has experienced symptoms of nausea and vomiting. Dr. Rice gives written orders to administer Imitrex 25 mg IM STAT, together with a prescription for the patient to fill and use at home. Lisa Cortes, CMA (AAMA), reviews the provider's order in Louise's medical record and prepares the STAT dosage for Louise according to the correct procedure for administering oral medications. Lisa is about to transport the medication to Louise in examination room 3 when she re-reads the provider's order for Louise, which calls for 25 mg IM STAT. The written prescription is for Imitrex every 4 hours as needed. Lisa discards the dosage she has prepared for the patient and instead gives Louise Dr. Rice's prescription and tells her to have it filled immediately.

CASE STUDY REVIEW QUESTIONS

1. What medication error has Lisa made? What effect will the error likely have on the patient?

____

____

____

____

2. What should Lisa have done? What standard procedures should be followed when a medication error occurs?

____

____

____

____

____

____

____

Reading Prescriptions

1. A prescription is a written legal document that gives directions for compounding, dispensing, and/or administering to a patient. Refer to the prescriptions shown below, and in the spaces provided, "decode" the prescriptions into lay terms and answer the questions that follow.

____

____

____

____

Dr. King prescribes an adult dosage for epilepsy.

INNER CITY HEALTH CARE
8600 MAIN STREET, SUITE 200
RIVER CITY, XY 01234

Name Lourdes Austin

Address 821 Spring Lane, Apt. 12 Date 3/1/XX

℞

Dilantin 100 mg tab
#90
Sig 100 mg p.o. tid

Generic Substitution Allowed Mark King M.D.
Dispense As Written M.D.
REFILL 0 1 2 3 p.r.n.
☑ LABEL

Dr. Lewis prescribes a child's dosage for an ear infection.

INNER CITY HEALTH CARE
8600 MAIN STREET, SUITE 200
RIVER CITY, XY 01234

Name Felicia Lawrence

Address 362 Owen's View Way Date 3/1/XX

℞

Amoxicillin 250 mg/5 mL.
#150 mL
Sig 500 mg p.o. tid

Generic Substitution Allowed Winston Lewis M.D.
Dispense As Written M.D.
REFILL 0 1 2 3 p.r.n.
☑ LABEL

2. How many grams are in each dose of Dilantin? ______
3. How many days of Dilantin are dispensed? ______
4. How many teaspoons are in 5 mL? ______
5. How many doses of amoxicillin are included in the amount dispensed? ______

ATTRIBUTES OF PROFESSIONALISM

1. Have you ever been given a shot? Do you remember how you felt just before the injection? Most people are more afraid of the pain of the injection than anything having to do with the medication. How can you utilize the Attributes of Professionalism in order to help your fearful patients feel less afraid? What could you do or say to alleviate their fears? Do you think only children are afraid of needles? Write down a couple of things you will do and say to help your patients. Discuss your ideas with a few classmates and listen to their ideas.

______
______
______
______
______

2. Write a step-by-step script regarding the preinjection instructions you would give to your patient, taking into account the Attributes of Professionalism.

Name ______________________ Date ________ Score ________

CHAPTER **36**

Cardiac Procedures

VOCABULARY BUILDER

Misspelled Words

From the following terms, find the misspelled words; circle them, and spell them correctly in the spaces provided. Then, fill in the blanks in the sentences below.

amplytude	deoxygenated	electrocardiography
cardiac catheterization	diastole	Halter monitor
cardiac cycle	electrocardigraph	isoelectic
defibrilation		

______________	______________	______________
______________	______________	______________

1. ______________ blood enters the right side of the heart.
2. The entire route of the electrical impulses through the heart is referred to as the ______________.
3. ______________ refers to the height of the ECG tracing.
4. Using an AED to restore a regular heart rhythm is called ______________.
5. The ______________ is a machine used to perform the ECG procedure.
6. The ______________ line is another name for the baseline on an ECG tracing.
7. The lowest amount of pressure on the vessel during a blood pressure reading is called ______________.
8. Ultrasonography and ______________ are noninvasive diagnostic procedures commonly used in the clinical setting.
9. The study of the coronary arteries using a radiopaque medium is called a ______________.
10. A ______________ is utilized to record heart rate and rhythm for a 24-hour period.

LEARNING REVIEW

Short answer

1. List five reasons why electrocardiography is performed.

____

____

____

____

____

2. The first three leads recorded on a standard ECG are leads I, II, and III. These leads are called _______________ leads because each of them uses two-limb electrodes that record simultaneously. For each lead, what electrical activity of the heart is recorded? Draw each lead's electrical activity on the corresponding figure.

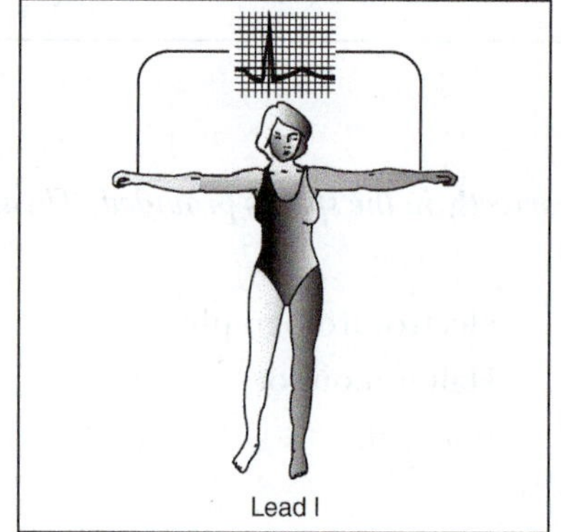
Lead I

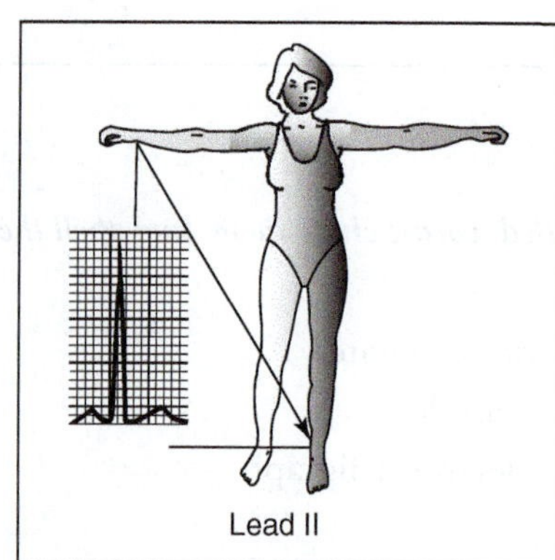
Lead II

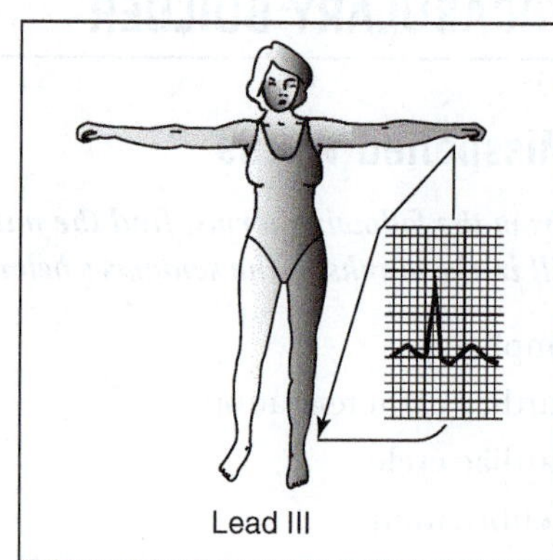
Lead III

3. Fill in the blanks:
   a. Lead I records electrical activity between the _______________ and the _______________.
   b. Lead II records electrical activity between the _______________ and the _______________.
   c. Lead III records electrical activity between the _______________ and the _______________.

4. The next group of leads recorded on a standard ECG are augmented leads, designated aV_R, aV_L, and aV_F. These are called _______________ leads. For each lead, what electrical activity of the heart is recorded? Draw each lead's electrical activity on the corresponding figure.

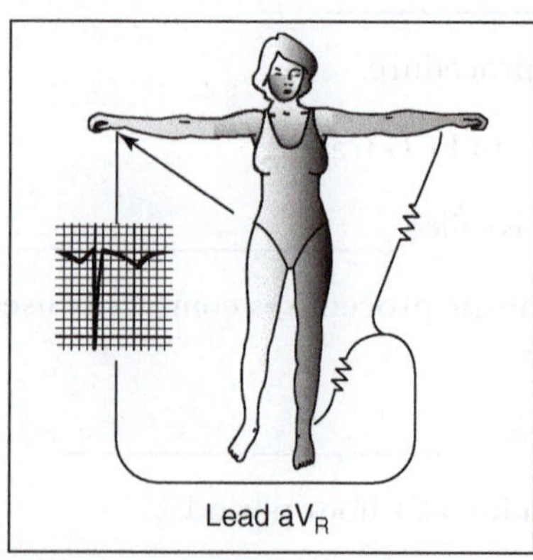
Lead aV_R

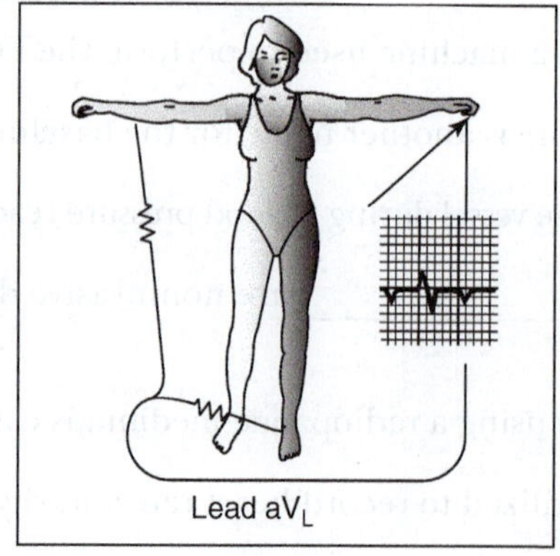
Lead aV_L

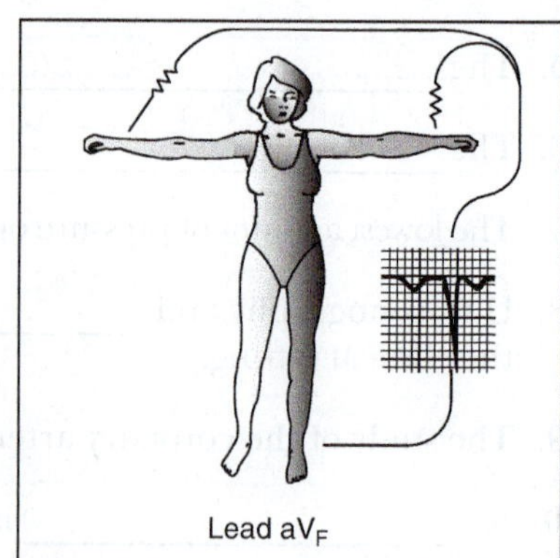
Lead aV_F

5. Fill in the blanks:

   a. Lead aV_R records electrical activity from the ______________________________ and the ______________________________.

   b. Lead aV_L records electrical activity from the ______________________________ and the ______________________________.

   c. Lead aV_F records electrical activity from the ______________________________ and the ______________________________.

6. The remaining 6 leads of the standard 12-lead ECG are called the chest leads, or precordial leads. These leads are (*circle the correct term*) unipolar/bipolar. Where are the leads placed on the body?

   V_1: ______________________________

   V_2: ______________________________

   V_3: ______________________________

   V_4: ______________________________

   V_5: ______________________________

   V_6: ______________________________

Identifying Artifact Activity

Artifacts are unusual and unwanted activity in the ECG tracing not caused by the electrical activity of the heart. Match each circumstance below to the artifact ECG tracing it would produce and identify the type of artifact in the space provided.

A. A broken patient cable or lead wire has become detached from an electrode.
B. The patient sings to himself during the ECG procedure.
C. The patient uses body lotion.
D. The lead wires are crossed and do not follow the patient's body contour.

	Type of Artifact	**Circumstance**
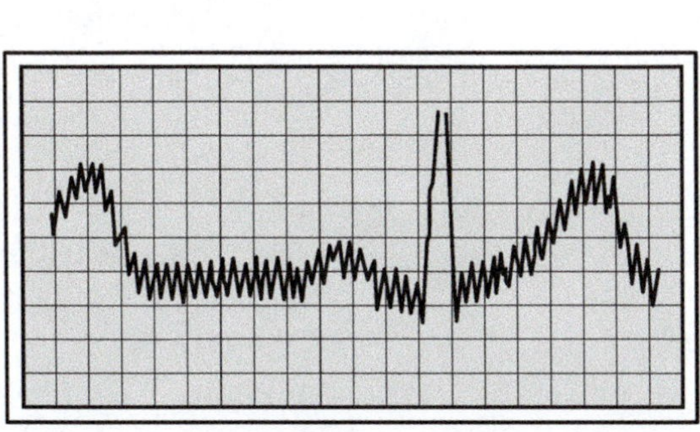	______________	____
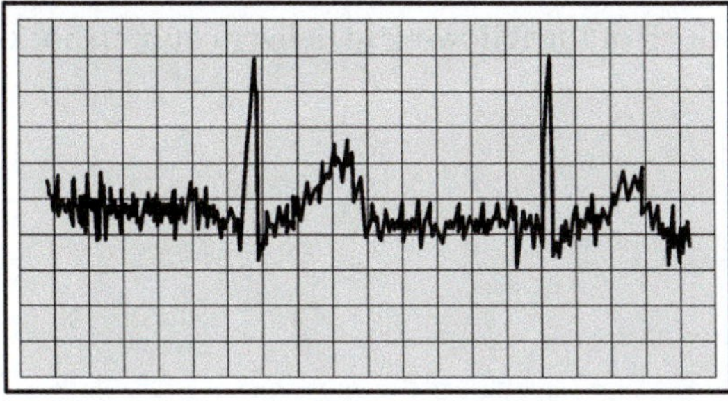	______________	____

Type of Artifact	Circumstance
____________	____
____________	____

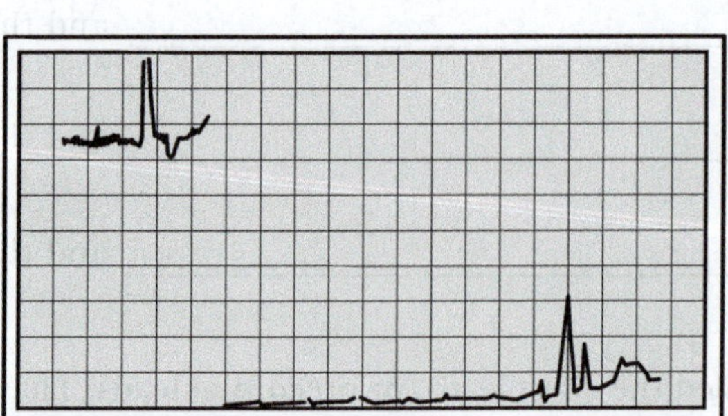

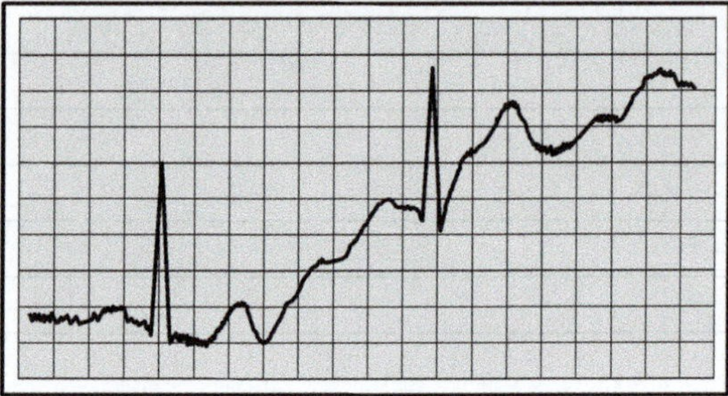

CERTIFICATION REVIEW

These questions are designed to mimic the certification examination. Select the best response.

1. What type of stress test is one in which the patient exercises on a treadmill after injection of a radioactive substance?
   a. Thallium
   b. Barium
   c. Nitrous oxide
   d. Bismuth

2. What is the name for chest leads?
   a. Precordial
   b. Limb
   c. Augmented
   d. Bipolar
   e. Unipolar

3. Treatment of life-threatening arrhythmias can be done using which of the following to deliver countershocks?
   a. Electrocardiograph
   b. Defibrillator
   c. Galvanometer
   d. Ultrasound

4. One millivolt of cardiac electrical activity will deflect the stylus how many millimeters in an upward direction?
   a. 5
   b. 10
   c. 25
   d. 40
   e. 50

5. A wandering baseline may be caused by which of the following?
   a. Lotions, creams, or oils on the patient's skin
   b. Electrical interference
   c. Crossed lead wires
   d. Improper grounding

6. Because the skin is a poor conductor of electricity, what substance is applied with each electrode?
   a. Electrolyte gel
   b. Adhesive
   c. Thallium
   d. Contrast
   e. Nitroglycerine

7. What is the name for a surgical procedure that takes a portion of a vein and grafts it to a coronary artery?
   a. Stenting
   b. Angioplasty
   c. Bypass
   d. Merging

8. A life-threatening arrhythmia in which the ventricles contract wildly is known as which of the following diagnoses?
   a. Premature ventricular contractions
   b. Ventricular fibrillation
   c. Ventricular tachycardia
   d. Sinus bradycardia
   e. Sinus tachycardia

9. Interference with the ECG tracing from other electrical sources is known as which of the following?
   a. Wandering baseline
   b. AC interference
   c. Arrhythmia
   d. Somatic tremor

10. A continuous record of cardiac activity for 24 hours or longer is provided by which device?
    a. ECG
    b. Holter monitor
    c. Defibrillator
    d. Echocardiograph
    e. AED

LEARNING APPLICATION

Critical Thinking

1. The provider wants you to explain to Mrs. Johnson (see Case Study 2 in core text) what behaviors she can adopt to have a healthy heart. With a partner, role play medical assistant and patient and explain to the patient what she can do to improve her heart's health.

2. Name four cardiac abnormalities that can be diagnosed using an ECG.

3. Identify the placement of the leads for a 12-lead ECG.

4. If a patient coughs or talks during an ECG, what effect will this have on the tracing?

Case Studies

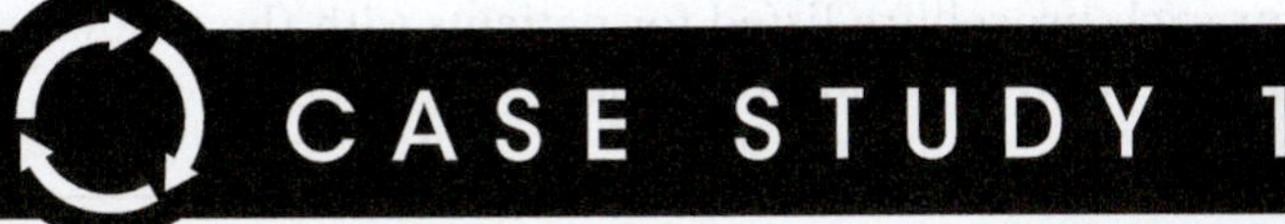

Jim Marshall, a prominent local architect in his late 30s, stays in good physical condition; works out regularly at the gym; and maintains a low-fat, low-cholesterol, low-sodium diet. Aggressive and ambitious, Jim enjoys pushing his mind and body to the limit. His favorite sports are skiing and sailing. At work, Jim is a perfectionist who puts in long hours and demands the same of his employees. Lately, though, Jim has been more aware of the high-stress lifestyle he is leading and is worried about his family history of heart failure and diabetes. During periods of high physical exertion, Jim experiences mild chest pain and palpitations. Dr. Lewis prescribes an exercise tolerance test for Jim.

CASE STUDY REVIEW QUESTIONS

1. What is an exercise tolerance test? How is it performed?

____

____

____

____

____

____

2. Under what conditions would the test be discontinued?

____

____

3. At the conclusion of the test, what patient care is given? What special instructions for home care should the patient observe?

____

____

____

Research Activities

Search the Internet for a national organization that focuses on heart and blood vessel disorders, such as the American Heart Association or the American College of Cardiology.

1. Print information about risk factors for cardiovascular heart disease.
2. What is the mortality rate for first-time myocardial infarctions for men versus women? Is there any difference in the mortality rate?
3. Are the symptoms identical in male and female patients when they are experiencing a myocardial infarction? Explain the similarities/differences between them.
4. Determine if there are newer types of 24-hour cardiac monitoring devices. How are they the same or different from the Holter monitor?

ATTRIBUTES OF PROFESSIONALISM

Write explanations regarding the rationale for each procedure listed for patients with the following levels of understanding—a medical professional and a person with no exposure to medical terms.

a. *Cardiac catheterization.* ______________________________

b. *Cardioversion.* ______________________________

c. *Defibrillation.* ______________________________

d. *Electrocardiogram.* ______________________________

e. *Holter monitor.* ______________________________

f. *Percutaneous transluminal coronary angioplasty (PTCA).* ______________________________

g. *Thallium stress testing.* ______________________________

h. *Cardiac ultrasonography.* ______________________________

Name ______________________ Date ________ Score ________

CHAPTER 37

Regulatory Guidelines for Safety and Quality in the Medical Laboratory

VOCABULARY BUILDER

Misspelled Words

Correct the spelling of the following terms and then define each term in the space provided.

1. Flume hoods ________ ______________________________

2. Liabel ________ ______________________________

3. Waved ________ ______________________________

Matching

Match each vocabulary term below with the correct definition in Column B.

	Column A	Column B
_____	1. Certificate of waiver	A. Describes a specimen that is easily broken down
_____	2. Labile	B. The process used to provide accurate, complete, consistent health care documentation in a timely manner while making every reasonable effort to resolve inconsistencies, inaccuracies, risk management issues, and other problems
_____	3. Proficiency testing	C. Describes a category of clinical laboratory tests that are simple, do not vary, and require a minimum of judgment and interpretation
_____	4. Waived	D. Measures used to monitor the processing of laboratory specimens

_____	5. Fume hoods	E.	Certificate issued to a laboratory to perform only waived tests
_____	6. Provider-performed microscopy procedures	F.	Sample tests performed in a clinical laboratory to determine that a specific degree of accuracy is achieved
_____	7. Quality assurance	G.	Written material provided by the manufacturer when chemicals are purchased; gives detailed information about the chemicals
_____	8. Safety Data Sheet	H.	A barrier used in the laboratory to capture chemical vapors
_____	9. Quality control	I.	CLIA term for microscopic examinations requiring at least a mid-level provider that has qualifications to perform the exam

LEARNING REVIEW

Short answer

1. CLIA '88 requires that every facility that tests human specimens for diagnosis, treatment, and prevention of disease meet specific federal requirements. Name four specific duties a medical assistant may perform that will impact the clinic's compliance with CLIA '88 regulations.

2. How does CLIA regulate quality control of automated hematology instruments?

3. What are the three categories of testing?

4. Describe the CMS 116 form and explain its purpose.

5. What are some personal safety precautions established by OSHA?

6. Why are SDSs important?

7. Name some unsafe working conditions and safety techniques that can be used to prevent accidents.

CERTIFICATION REVIEW

These questions are designed to mimic the certification examination. Select the best response.

1. What is the purpose of CLIA?
   a. To teach staff how to read test results accurately
   b. To establish standards to ensure the confidentiality of test results
   c. To safeguard the public by regulating all testing of specimens taken from the human body
   d. All of the above

2. CLIA was passed in what year?
   a. 1902
   b. 1975
   c. 1988
   d. 1999
   e. 2001

3. Which of the following procedures is a requirement of qualifying protocol for automated hematology instruments?
   a. Control samples
   b. Proficiency testing
   c. Calibration
   d. All of the above

4. Of the following choices, what do Safety Data Sheets (SDSs) *not* contain?
   a. Product/chemical information
   b. Emergency response procedures
   c. Manufacturer information
   d. Training information related to using the product/chemical
   e. Reactivity data

5. When skin comes into contact with chemicals, what is best practice?
   a. Wash the area with water immediately
   b. Apply a neutralizing agent to the site
   c. Consult the SDS before treatment
   d. Rinse area with vinegar

6. Which federal agency oversees the safety of health facilities, including protection against occupational hazards such as bloodborne pathogens?
   a. OSHA
   b. CLIA'88
   c. FDA
   d. CDC
   e. EPA

7. Which of the following laboratory tests are not PPMP levels of testing?
   a. Urine sediment examinations
   b. Qualitative semen analysis
   c. Urine pregnancy test
   d. Wet mount preparations

8. Which professionals obtain specific formal training in waived category testing procedures?
   a. Physicians
   b. Registered nurses
   c. Medical technicians
   d. Medical assistants
   e. All of the above

9. If any lab changes the type of tests it performs, the lab must contact the CMS within what amount of time?
   a. 1 month
   b. 2 months
   c. 6 months
   d. 1 year

10. What issuing agency established the guidelines for Standard Precautions?
    a. OSHA
    b. DHHS
    c. CMS
    d. FDA
    e. CDC

LEARNING APPLICATION

Critical Thinking

1. Explain the purpose of CLIA '88 and why the law was amended.

___

___

___

2. Describe quality control and quality assurance. Why are they important?

___

___

___

___

___

___

___

3. You have been asked to develop a manual for your provider-employer. The manual is to detail a chemical hygiene plan (CHP) for all employees in the office. How would you proceed? What should be included in the plan? In the CHP, include three major goals that will ensure the provider-employer's compliance with the hazard standard.

4. You have been asked to compile a manual of the SDSs for chemicals used in your workplace. What must be included in the manual and from where does the information come?

ATTRIBUTES OF PROFESSIONALISM

There is much to think about when it comes to safety in the clinic. As a medical assistant, you must have a heightened awareness for the safety of the patient as well as yourself. Write in your journal how you would react, incorporating the Attributes of Professionalism, to one of the following regulatory or safety issues: needlestick, chemical splash in your eyes, misreading a waived test result, or using expired reagents.

Think about chemicals you have in your home. Does the information you have learned in this chapter make you more aware and perhaps want to take a second look? Choose a chemical that is hazardous. Take a look at the label(s). Does it have any precautionary warnings? Does it have any fire hazard information? What changes, if any, to the way you handle and store chemicals would you make? What is the number in your area for Poison Control?

Name ______________________ Date ________ Score ________

CHAPTER 38

Introduction to the Medical Laboratory

VOCABULARY BUILDER

Misspelled Words

Find the words below that are misspelled; circle them, and correctly spell them in the space provided.

control test	clinical diagnosis	quantative tests
baseline values	differential diagnosis	regents
biopsy	qualitative tests	requasition
____________	____________	____________

Fill in the Blanks

From the list above, insert the correct vocabulary terms into the sentences below. Each sentence describes a situation you might find in a POL or in a reference laboratory.

1. Dr. Angie Osborne orders laboratory tests for a female patient experiencing severe abdominal cramps in order to make a ____________ that will distinguish between a diagnosis of appendicitis and a diagnosis of an ovarian cyst.

2. Richard Butts receives a job offer from a construction company that requires all employees to be tested for general overall health before they can work at the site. Gwen Carr, CMA (AAMA), performs Richard's blood test under the direction of Dr. Lewis; his test comes back within normal limits. The results of Richard's test can be used in the future as ____________, a record of healthy normal results.

3. Dr. King needs a red blood cell (RBC) count, a white blood cell (WBC) count, and a platelet count for Melinda Cool. Joe Guerrero, CMA (AAMA), performs a venipuncture on Melinda and sends a tube of her blood to the laboratory, together with a written ____________ containing specific information and instructions about what tests to perform on the specimens.

4. Hematology laboratories count the WBCs and RBCs in a sample of a patient's blood. In general, these types of counting tests with numerical results are known as ____________.

5. As a method of quality control, a ______________________ sample is tested together with a patient's sample as a method of ensuring the accuracy of test results.

6. The hematology laboratory performs tests that measure characteristics of blood such as size, shape, and maturity of cells. These types of tests are known in general as ______________________.

7. Histology is the study of tissue samples to determine disease. In most cases, a tissue sample or ______________________ is frozen, sliced, stained, and microscopically examined for anomalies.

8. If a control sample shows inaccurate results after testing, one possible explanation is that the ______________________ are faulty or have expired.

9. A ______________________ of Lyme disease can be confirmed by performing laboratory tests on patient blood specimens.

LEARNING REVIEW

Matching

Match each category of laboratory test to the phrase below that best fits it.

A. Clinical chemistry

B. Cytology

C. Hematology

D. Histology

E. Serology (immunology/immunohematology) and blood banking

F. Parasitology

G. Microbiology

H. Urinalysis

______ 1. Prothrombin time (PT)

______ 2. Alkaline phosphatase (APT)

______ 3. Color, clarity, specific gravity

______ 4. C-reactive protein test (CRP)

______ 5. Platelet count

______ 6. Toxoplasmosis

______ 7. Creatinine

______ 8. Tapeworm disease (enterobiasis)

______ 9. Tissue analysis

______ 10. Pap test

______ 11. Chlamydia

______ 12. Mono test

Short Answer

1. Identify each abbreviated test named below.

Hgb	
Diff	
ESR	
Hct	
O&P	

2. Name three criteria that would justify using point-of-care testing.

3. What is the reason for using a control test sample? Explain in detail.

4. Name the five parts of a microscope.

5. What type of microscope is most commonly used in a medical laboratory?

6. Name three other types of microscopes and explain what each is designed for viewing.

7. Name the two adjustments found on a microscope and explain the purpose of each.

8. Name six practices that should always be followed to properly care for a microscope.

CERTIFICATION REVIEW

These questions are designed to mimic the certification examination. Select the best response.

1. Choosing to perform the simplest and least invasive procedure to rule out a particular disease before requiring more extensive testing is known as what?
   a. Obtaining a clinical diagnosis
   b. Obtaining a cumulative diagnosis
   c. Obtaining a developmental diagnosis
   d. Obtaining a differential diagnosis

2. What type of test involves actual number counts such as are done in WBC counts, RBC counts, and platelet levels?
   a. Qualitative tests
   b. Quantitative tests
   c. CLIA-waived tests
   d. Functional tests
   e. Cytology tests

3. The category of lab test that best describes what is used to test tetanus, gonorrhea, tuberculosis, and pertussis is called what?
   a. Cytology
   b. Chemistry
   c. Microbiology
   d. Histology

4. A hepatic function panel will include which of the following?
   a. Creatinine level
   b. Rheumatoid factor
   c. Cholesterol level
   d. Bilirubin level
   e. Sodium level

5. Analysis of abnormal tissue cells such as chromosome studies is known as which of the following?
   a. Hematology
   b. Serology
   c. Microbiology
   d. Cytology

6. Which of the following panel tests are ordered for diagnostic testing on the liver?
   a. Hepatic function panel
   b. Arthritis panel
   c. Renal function panel
   d. Cholesterol screening panel
   e. Thyroid function panel

7. Many clinics require that pending lab reports contained within the EMR are to be reviewed and signed by a provider within what length of time?
   a. 6 to 12 hours
   b. 12 to 24 hours
   c. 24 to 36 hours
   d. 36 to 48 hours

8. By what other name is POCT testing often referred to as?
   a. Patient office care testing
   b. Bedside testing
   c. At home testing
   d. Pharmacy testing
   e. Rapid testing

9. During a physical examination, what are healthy or normal test results also known as?
   a. Metabolic level
   b. Calibration level
   c. Reference ranges
   d. None of the above

10. If a TDM specimen is drawn 30 minutes after the last dosage of medication was given to a patient, what would you be testing for?
    a. Trough level
    b. Random level
    c. Peak level
    d. Toxicity
    e. Reference level

LEARNING APPLICATION

Critical Thinking

1. A patient asks you to recommend a laboratory for the tests ordered by the provider. How will you respond to the request? What are some factors that will influence your response?

____

____

____

____

2. A patient performed a pregnancy test at home, but her provider has requested a pregnancy test at the clinic. How will you explain to the patient why the home test may not be as accurate as the test performed at the clinic?

____

____

____

____

Case Studies

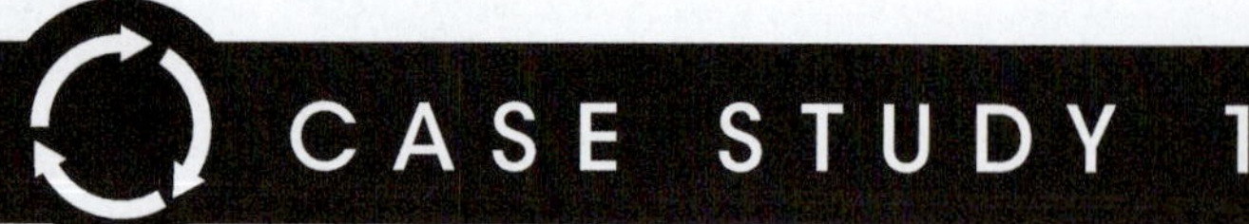

You come to work one morning to discover the electricity has gone off in the refrigerator in the laboratory. This refrigerator houses the reagents needed to perform the laboratory tests.

CASE STUDY REVIEW QUESTIONS

1. How will you proceed?

____

____

____

____

____

2. Is there a way to determine whether or not the reagents are still acceptable?

____

____

____

3. How could this have been prevented?

____

____

____

____

____

____

Hands-on Activity

At Abigail Johnson's annual physical examination on June 5, 20XX, at 2 PM, Dr. Mark King orders several laboratory tests to monitor Abigail's diagnosed conditions of hypertension, diabetes mellitus, and moderate angina pectoris. Dr. Frank Jones, Abigail's cardiologist, will also receive a copy of the final laboratory report. Gwen Carr, CMA (AAMA), begins to prepare the laboratory requisition form. Complete Gwen's laboratory requisition form for Abigail's laboratory work.

Patient:	Physician:
Abigail Johnson 225 River Street River City, XY 01234 Phone: 389-2631 Date of Birth: March 1, 1940 Social Security Number: 011-11-1231 Medicare #: 021-45-6712-D	Dr. Mark King Inner City Health Care 8600 Main Street, Suite 200 River City, XY 01234 Phone: 456-7890 Dr. Frank Jones 815 Heart Health Blvd River City, XY 01234 Phone: 655-7000

Physician's Order for Laboratory Testing: Blood panel to include BUN, chloride, cholesterol, creatinine, glucose, LDH, potassium, SGOT (AST), SGPT (ALT), sodium, and triglycerides.

BILL ☐ ACCOUNT ☐ PATIENT SEE ① ☐ 3RD PARTY SEE ②	PLEASE LEAVE BLANK AREA DEPT. BILL CD	C-3 REQUEST FORM INSTRUCTIONS ① FOR PATIENT BILLING, COMPLETE BOX A ② FOR 3RD PARTY BILLING, COMPLETE BOX A AND FILL IN DIAGNOSIS, THEN EITHER B, C, OR D	USA Labs 957 Main Street Heartland, NY 11112

PATIENT NAME (LAST) (FIRST)	SPECIES	SEX	AGE YRS. MOS.	DATE COLLECTED MO. DAY YR.	TIME COLLECTED
PATIENT ADDRESS STREET	MISC. INFORMATION		DR. I.D.	MEDICARE #	
CITY STATE ZIP	DIAGNOSIS				
PHYSICIAN	WELFARE: #		CASE NAME:		
	PROGRAM:	PATIENT 1ST NAME:	DATE OF BIRTH ALL CLAIMS	MO. DAY YR.	
	INSURANCE GR. #	I.D.	SERVICE CODE:		
	SUBSCRIBER NAME:		RELATION:	PHONE	

Standard Profiles

Code		Profile	Code		Profile
2987	()	Diagnostic (Multi-Chem) Profile	8350	()	Immunologic Evaluation*
2804	()	Health Survey (SMA-12)	2814	()	Lipid Profile A
2824	()	Executive Profile A	2817	()	Lipid Profile B
2825	()	Executive Profile B	2003	()	Lipid Profile C
2826	()	Executive Profile C	2805	()	Liver Profile A
2858	()	Amenorrhea Profile	2867	()	Liver Profile B
7330	()	Anticonvulsant Group	2868	()	MMR Immunity Panel
2927	()	Autoimmune Profile	2869	()	Myocardial Infarction Profile
2801	()	Calcium Metabolism Profile	2585	()	Parathyroid Panel A (Mid-Molecule)
2859	()	Diabetes Management Profile	2586	()	Parathyroid Panel B (Dialysis)
7701	()	Drug Abuse Screen	2587	()	Parathyroid Panel C (Adenoma)
	()	Drug Analysis Comprehensive (S & U or G)	2818	()	Prenatal Profile A
			2819	()	Prenatal Profile B
	()	Drug Analysis, Qual (U/G)	2820	()	Prenatal Profile C
7340	()	Drug Analysis, Quant. (S)	2877	()	Prenatal Profile D
2022	()	Electrolyte Profile		()	Respiratory Infection Profile A
	()	Exanthem Group		()	Respiratory Infection Profile B
	()	Glucose/Insulin Response		()	Respiratory Infection Profile C
2871	()	Hepatitis Profile I		()	Respiratory Infection Profile D
2872	()	Hepatitis Profile II	2821	()	Rheumatoid Profile A
2873	()	Hepatitis Profile III	2878	()	Rheumatoid Profile B
2874	()	Hepatitis Profile IV	2882	()	T & B Lymphocyte Differential Panel
2875	()	Hepatitis Profile V			
2876	()	Hepatitis Profile VI	2883	()	Testicular Function Profile
2879	()	Hepatitis Profile VII	2832	()	Thyroid Panel A
2864	()	Hirsutism Profile	2032	()	Thyroid Panel B
2865	()	Hypertension Screen	2833	()	Thyroid Panel C

Single Tests

Code		Test	Code		Test
5165	()	ABO and Rho (B) (S)	6526	()	Neonatal T_4 (S)
6555	()	Alpha-Fetoprotein RIA (S)	6525	()	Neonatal TSH (S)
3015	()	Alk. Phosphatase (s)	7941	()	Neonatal Tf Blood Spot
3041	()	Amylase (S)	3019	()	Phosphorus (S)
5163	()	Antibody Screen () If pos. ID & Titer (S) (B)	4132	()	Platelet Count (B) (S)
5166	()	Antibody ID (B&S)	3026	()	Potassium (S)
5164	()	Antibody Titer (B&S)		()	Pregnancy Test, (S or U)
		(Previous Pat. #__________)	5187	()	Premarital RPR (S)
5208	()	ANA. Flourescent (S)	6505	()	Prostatic Acid Phosphatase (RIA) (S)*
5169	()	ASO Titer (B) (S)			
3147	()	Bilirubin, Direct (S)	2992	()	Protein Electrophoresis (S)
3010	()	BUN (S)			IEP if Abnormal () 9085
3018	()	Calcium (S)	4149	()	Prothrombin Time (P)*
6472	()	CEA (RIA) (Plasma Only)	4144	()	Reticulocyte Count (B)
2995	()	CBC with Automated Diff.	5207	()	RA Latex Fixation (s)
		(Abnormal Follow-Up Studies) (B)(SL)	5194	()	RPR
2996	()	CBC less Diff. (B)	5195	()	Rubella H.I. (S)
3022	()	Cholesterol (S)	3016	()	SGOT (S)
3042	()	CPK (S)	3045	()	SGPT (S)
6500	()	Digoxin (S)	3031	()	T-3 Uptake (S)
6501	()	Digitoxin (S)	3032	()	T-4 (S)
3606	()	GGT (S)	2832	()	Thyroxine Index, Free (T_7) (S)
3006	()	Glucose (S) Fasting	3036	()	Truglycerides
3009	()	Glucose (P) Fasting	4111	()	Urinalysis (U)
3023	()	Glucose P.P. (P) Hrs. __________	5277	()	Urogenital GC Assay
3650	()	HDL Cholesterol (S)			UNLISTED TESTS OR PROFILES
5180	()	Heterophile Screen (Mono) (S)			
5179	()	Hererophile Absorption (S)			
3342	()	Hemoglobin A_{1C} (B)			
6416	()	IgE (S)			
3078	()	Iron and T.I.B.C. (S)			

* FROZEN • (B) BLOOD • (P) PLASMA • (U) URINE • (S) SERUM • (SL) SLIDES

FOLD THIS FORM IN HALF SO TEST(S) ORDERED IS CLEARLY VISIBLE

ATTRIBUTES OF PROFESSIONALISM

Working in a medical laboratory requires spending a significant amount of time performing extremely detail-oriented procedures, such as observing specimens through a microscope for signs of disease. Laboratory analysis also involves maintaining high-quality controls and safety standards to ensure the accuracy and reliability of results. The way you deal with details in your everyday life can reveal much about your predisposition for detail-oriented analytic tasks.

Write in your journal how the Attributes of Professionalism will apply to your work in a medical laboratory. Take into consideration both your personal and professional life experiences. Describe a particular area of interest or experience you may have regarding laboratory testing.

Name ______________________ Date ________ Score ________

CHAPTER 39

Phlebotomy: Venipuncture and Capillary Puncture

VOCABULARY BUILDER

Misspelled Words

Find the words listed below that are misspelled; circle them, and correctly spell them in the spaces provided. Then match each vocabulary term with the correct definition below.

additive	hemotoma	thirotrophic gel
aliquet	palpatate	thrombocyte
hemoconcentration	plasma	venipuncture
hemololysis	serum	

______________ ______________ ______________

______________ ______________ ______________

1. ______________ The fluid portion of blood from an anticoagulated blood collection tube
2. ______________ The process of collecting blood
3. ______________ A portion of a blood sample that has been taken off for use or storage
4. ______________ Any material placed in a blood collection tube that maintains or facilitates the integrity and function of the specimen
5. ______________ To feel, as in feeling for a vein
6. ______________ An accumulation of blood around the venipuncture site during or after venipuncture, caused by leakage of blood from where the needle punctured the vein
7. ______________ The destruction of blood in a sample; the rupture of the red blood cells
8. ______________ The fluid portion of the blood after clotting has taken place

9. ____________________ A gel material capable of forming an interface between the cells and fluid portion of the blood sample as a result of centrifugation

10. ____________________ Platelet

11. ____________________ Occurs when a tourniquet is left on the arm longer than 1 minute, causing an increased concentration of constituents in the blood sample, resulting in inaccurate test results

LEARNING REVIEW

Short Answer

1. Identify and describe the first-, second-, and third-choice sites used to perform venipuncture on the human body.

____

____

____

____

____

____

2. Tourniquets play a critical role in venipuncture and must be applied and used properly to obtain a blood specimen for analysis.

   A. What is the purpose of a tourniquet?

   ____

   ____

   B. Where is the tourniquet placed?

   ____

   ____

   C. How long should the tourniquet remain on the arm during the procedure?

   ____

   ____

   D. At what point during the procedure should the tourniquet be removed? Why is the timing of removal so important?

   ____

   ____

   ____

3. Match the collection tubes containing anticoagulants with their corresponding color stoppers: green, gray, blue, and lavender.

   A. Coagulation citrate tube: ________

   B. EDTA tube: ________

   C. Glycolytic inhibitor tube: ________

   D. Heparin tube: ________

4. Vein stimulation refers to techniques used when initial attempts to obtain a blood sample are not successful. List five techniques used to stimulate veins.

____

____

____

____

____

5. Describe the characteristics of a vein versus an artery versus a tendon when palpating and drawing blood.

____

____

____

6. Identify the recommended venipuncture method for each of the situations listed below.
   A. When drawing blood from a 75-year-old patient with thin veins _______________
   B. When collecting a blood specimen a child, who has small veins and a tendency to move during the venipuncture procedure _______________
   C. When multiple blood samples must be obtained from one venipuncture procedure _______________

7. What are two of the most common reactions patients have during venipuncture?

____

____

8. In preparing a patient for venipuncture, why would it be helpful to know about the patient's past venipuncture experiences?

____

____

____

____

9. Why does the appearance and attitude of the medical assistant matter when approaching a patient for a blood sample?

____

____

____

Matching

Arteries and veins are crucial elements of the circulatory system. Indicate which of the following are functions or characteristics of arteries (A) and which are functions of veins (V).

_______ 1. Blood is brighter in color

_______ 2. No pulse

_______ 3. Thin and fragile

CERTIFICATION REVIEW

These questions are designed to mimic the certification examination. Select the best response.

1. What machine uses force to push the blood clot to the bottom of the tube, leaving the clear serum on top?
   a. Autoclave
   b. Centrifuge
   c. Calibrator
   d. Incubator

2. What does plasma contain that differs from serum?
   a. Fibrinogen
   b. A buffy coat
   c. RBCs
   d. A clot
   e. WBCs

3. What is the correct needle position to be inserted for venipuncture?
   a. 90 degrees
   b. 30 degrees
   c. 45 degrees
   d. 15 degrees

4. What is the first step in a successful venipuncture?
   a. Select the site
   b. Put the patient at ease
   c. Apply the tourniquet appropriately
   d. Apply gloves
   e. Label the tubes with patient name

5. What is another term for syncope?
   a. Fasting
   b. Relaxation
   c. Fainting
   d. Reclining

6. Certain levels of blood components are decreased in capillaries. Which of the following is not decreased?
   a. Potassium
   b. Total protein
   c. Calcium
   d. Glucose
   e. None of the above

7. Which of the following additives does not bind with calcium when mixed with the blood specimen?
   a. Sodium fluoride
   b. Potassium oxalate
   c. Sodium citrate
   d. EDTA

8. What is a buffy coat?
   a. Heavier erythrocytes
   b. Plasma
   c. Hemoglobin
   d. A mixture of leukocytes and thrombocytes
   e. Both a and c

9. Where are red blood cells (RBCs) produced?
   a. Liver
   b. Lymph nodes
   c. Spleen
   d. Bone marrow

10. What is the most common size needle used for regular vacuum tube systems?
    a. 16 G
    b. 18 G
    c. 20 G
    d. 21 G
    e. 22 G

LEARNING APPLICATION

Critical Thinking

1. Explain the difference between serum and plasma. Describe how serum and plasma samples are collected.

2. How can vein collapse be avoided in a geriatric patient?

3. Discuss how clots are formed and what can be done to stop the clotting process.

4. The patient cries out in pain when you insert the needle into the vein. What will you do to make the patient more comfortable? If you decide to try another site, how will you locate it?

Case Studies

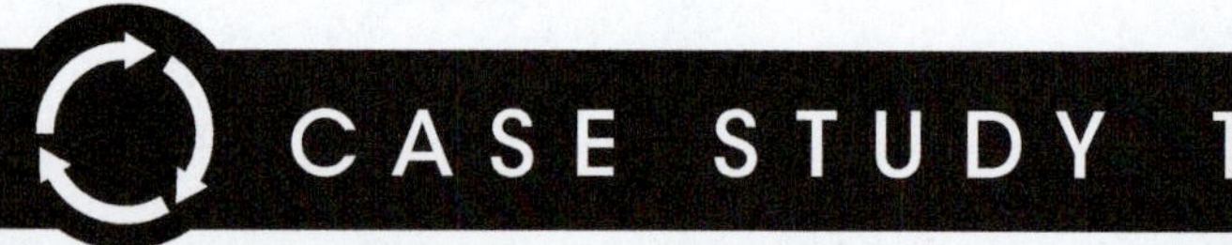

Nancy McFarland, RMA (AMT), performs a successful venipuncture on Jaime Carrera using the vacuum tube system and a 21-G needle. Nancy is now preparing to label the tubes for laboratory analysis. She is careful to label all tubes at the patient's side before leaving the examination room.

CASE STUDY REVIEW QUESTIONS

1. What information must be included on the specimen labels for the specimen to be accepted for analysis?

2. What guidelines must Nancy follow during the venipuncture procedure to ensure that anticoagulated blood specimens are acceptable for analysis?

3. Once Nancy has followed all procedures for collecting the blood specimens, what safety precautions must she perform?

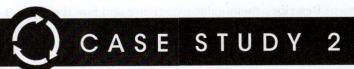

After you have drawn two tubes of blood and the patient has left, you drop one of the tubes and it breaks, scattering glass and splashing blood all over the area. Fortunately, this area is not in the main traffic flow of the clinic.

CASE STUDY REVIEW QUESTIONS

1. How do you proceed?

____

____

____

____

____

____

2. Could this accident have been prevented?

____

____

____

Hands-on Activities

Make your own flashcards using the form on the last page of this chapter. Tear out the page of flashcards and copy them double-sided onto a cardstock or heavy-weight paper. Cut them apart. Color in the "O" with the same color as the vacuum tube tops (brick red, lavender, green, blue, etc.) and fill in the information. Use the cards to drill yourself and your classmates.

ATTRIBUTES OF PROFESSIONALISM

1. During your career as a medical assistant, you will most likely run into a patient who refuses to have his or her blood drawn. Referring to the Attributes of Professionalism, think about the following:
   - How will you calm the patient?
   - What measures might you take that may be different from those used during typical blood draws?
   - What would make you decide not to continue with a blood draw?
   - How would you chart each situation?

____

____

2. How do you feel about having blood drawn? Describe a memorable experience and how the medical assistant or phlebotomist made the experience better or worse. Now apply the Attributes of Professionalism and write in your journal about how you would handle performing venipuncture and capillary puncture. How does your personal experience as a patient influence your actions?

O	Color: Additive: Specimen type: Tests:
O	Color: Additive: Specimen type: Tests:
O	Color: Additive: Specimen type: Tests:
O	Color: Additive: Specimen type: Tests:
O	Color: Additive: Specimen type: Tests:
O	Color: Additive: Specimen type: Tests:
O	Color: Additive: Specimen type: Tests:
O	Color: Additive: Specimen type: Tests:

Name ______________________ Date ________ Score ________

CHAPTER 40

Hematology

VOCABULARY BUILDER

Misspelled Words

Find the words in Column A that are misspelled; circle them, and correctly spell them in the spaces provided. Then match each vocabulary term below in Column A with the correct definition in Column B.

	Column A	Correct Spelling	Column B
_____	1. Complete blood count	____________	A. A hormone produced by the kidneys that helps with RBC production
_____	2. Erythrocysts	____________	B. Having less color than normal
_____	3. Esinophils	____________	C. A larger than normal cell
_____	4. Microcytic	____________	D. A WBC without cytoplasmic granules; has a large, convoluted, nonsegmented nucleus
_____	5. Luekocytes	____________	E. A smaller than normal cell
_____	6. Hematacrit	____________	F. WBCs, one of the formed elements of blood
_____	7. Hemaglobin	____________	G. WBC with a dense, nonsegmented nucleus that lacks granules in the cytoplasm
_____	8. Basophils	____________	H. Platelets
_____	9. Thrombocytes	____________	I. Granulocytic WBC with dark purple cytoplasmic granules
_____	10. Lymphocyte	____________	J. Molecule of the RBC that transports oxygen
_____	11. Monocytes	____________	K. Test to measure the percentage of RBCs within a specimen of anticoagulated whole blood
_____	12. Macrocytic	____________	L. A granulocytic WBC with red-stained granules in the cytoplasm; is increased with allergies
_____	13. Hypochromic	____________	M. RBCs, one of the formed elements of blood
_____	14. Erythropotin	____________	N. Hematologic test consisting of Hct, Hgb, RBC and WBC counts, differential WBC count, and erythrocyte indices

LEARNING REVIEW

Short Answer

1. When Dr. Winston Lewis orders CBCs on his patients, what are the general tests the provider will study to help him make a diagnosis?

2. While Dr. Mark King is reviewing blood tests drawn on one of his patients, he notes the hematocrit is normal, yet the hemoglobin is low. This is an indication of which disease?

3. Identify and explain the following erythrocyte indices:

   MCH:

   MCHC:

   MCV:

4. Sedimentation rate results vary with different states of health. Name two factors that influence sedimentation rate. Why is the ESR a more accurate tool in diagnosing the onset of a disease than in checking on the progress of treatment?

5. At Inner City Health Care, Gwen Carr, CMA (AAMA), uses automated hematology instruments. Automated hematology procedures have many advantages over manual methods. List five of these advantages.

6. Define hematopoiesis and describe where hematopoiesis occurs from the embryo through adulthood.

Matching

Match the appropriate adult parameters with the corresponding blood tests.

_____ 1. 50 to 55% — A. Normal hemoglobin value for adult male

_____ 2. 80 to 100 fL — B. Leukocyte count for an adult

_____ 3. 4,500 to 11,000/mm^3 — C. Normal mean corpuscular volume

_____ 4. 32 to 36 g/dL — D. Normal hematocrit value for adult male

_____ 5. 4.0 to 5.5 × 10^6/mm^3 — E. Normal mean corpuscular hemoglobin

_____ 6. 13 to 18 g/dL — F. Normal erythrocyte count for adult female

_____ 7. 27 to 33 pg — G. Normal value for MCHC

CERTIFICATION REVIEW

These questions are designed to mimic the certification examination. Select the best response.

1. What is the central component of each heme group?
   a. Magnesium
   b. Calcium
   c. Potassium
   d. Iron molecule

2. A buffy coat contains WBCs and which of the following?
   a. RBCs
   b. Plasma
   c. Platelets
   d. Serum
   e. All of the above

3. When a patient has RBCs with less hemoglobin content (hypochromic), what disease does he or she have?
   a. Hyperchromic disease
   b. Iron deficiency anemia
   c. Polychromic disease
   d. Bichromic disease

4. Increased eosinophils may indicate what condition/disease?
   a. Hay fever or other allergic conditions
   b. Leukemia
   c. Appendicitis
   d. Tuberculosis
   e. HIV

5. Hematocrit (packed RBC volume) is the ratio of the volume of packed RBCs to which of the following?
   a. The whole-blood specimen
   b. Leukocytes
   c. Thrombocytes
   d. All of the above

6. Which leukocyte is the most numerous within the body?
   a. Eosinophils
   b. Neutrophils
   c. Lymphocytes
   d. Monocytes
   e. Buffy coat

7. What are erythrocytes of normal size called?
   a. Erythrocytic
   b. Normocytic
   c. Macrocytic
   d. Microcytic

8. Erythropoietin is produced where in the body?
   a. Spleen
   b. Kidneys
   c. Bone marrow
   d. Pancreas
   e. Liver

9. Manual blood cell counts are considered by the Clinical Laboratory Improvement Act (CLIA) to be of what complexity?
   a. Waived
   b. Moderate to high
   c. High
   d. PPMP

10. What is the most common type of anemia found in a clinical setting?
    a. Iron-deficiency anemia
    b. Hemorrhagic anemia
    c. Aplastic anemia
    d. Nutritional anemia
    e. HIV

LEARNING APPLICATION

Critical Thinking

1. What hematologic factors do erythrocyte indices provide information about? List one example for each index in which a disease causes an elevation or decrease.

2. You are doing your practicum in a local clinic. A provider has made a tentative diagnosis of appendicitis for a patient. In addition to the urinalysis, what single hematologic test is most likely to confirm the diagnosis?

3. What test would have elevated results if a patient had lupus? Why?

Case Studies

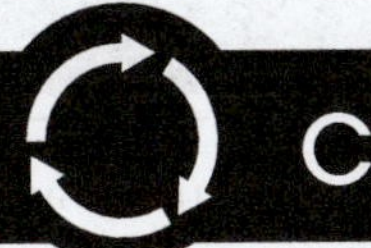

CASE STUDY 1

Jackson Tyndall is a regular patient at Inner City Health Care. Two days ago, he began to feel fatigued and developed a cough, fever, and chills. Dr. Reynolds has examined Mr. Tyndall and, based on the presenting symptoms, makes a clinical diagnosis of influenza.

CASE STUDY REVIEW QUESTIONS

1. What type of blood test might Dr. Reynolds order to confirm his diagnosis?

2. What type of results are to be expected based on a diagnosis confirming clinical data?

CASE STUDY 2

Mary Manning is describing a constant rundown feeling. After examining her, Dr. Mark King orders a hemoglobin determination and a thyroid panel. Also, because of a past history of a blood transfusion, he has ordered an HIV test to be done at an outside reference laboratory. Dr. King asks Joe Guerrero, CMA (AAMA), to perform the venipuncture procedure on Mary to obtain the blood specimens for analysis.

CASE STUDY REVIEW QUESTIONS

1. What tube will Joe use to collect the blood sample to be used for the hemoglobin determination test?

2. What is Dr. King hoping to learn from the hemoglobin test results?

3. Because HIV infection cannot yet be ruled out, what Standard Precautions should Joe follow in performing the venipuncture and the automated hemoglobin determination test?

CASE STUDY 3

During an ESR test, the rack that is holding the filled tubes is bumped and the entire rack, tubes and all, is knocked over. Fortunately, the tubes are securely capped so no blood has spilled.

CASE STUDY REVIEW QUESTIONS

1. Can you proceed with the test or must it be redone?

2. Could this accident have been prevented?

ATTRIBUTES OF PROFESSIONALISM

Hematology is the study of the blood cells and coagulation in both normal and diseased states. How would you apply the Attributes of Professionalism to what you learned in this chapter? Consider any personal feelings about performing venipuncture and testing blood. Do you think you will be more cautious with a patient who has HIV than with one who does not? Why or why not? Do you think you should be notified if the blood you are drawing or testing is known to be HIV positive? Do you have the same concerns with hepatitis-infected specimens? Explain your rationale and cite examples of how you would exhibit Attributes of Professionalism when performing venipuncture and testing blood.

Name________________________ Date__________ Score__________

CHAPTER 41

Urinalysis

VOCABULARY BUILDER

Misspelled Words

Find the words in Column A that are misspelled; circle them, and then correctly spell them in the spaces provided. Then match each vocabulary term below with the correct definition in Column B.

	Column A	Correct Spelling	Column B
____	1. Ketones	________	A. 24-hour period of waking and sleeping
____	2. pH	________	B. Crystalline material found in urine sediment; shapeless; possessing no definite form
____	3. Sedament	________	C. Compounds produced during increased fat metabolism; can be tested on a reagent strip
____	4. Amorphus	________	D. The burning of fats for energy
____	5. Casts	________	E. The liquid (top) portion of centrifuged urine that is disposed of
____	6. Sircadium rithm	________	F. An infection of the urinary system
____	7. Specific gravity	________	G. Scale that indicates the relative alkalinity or acidity of a solution; measurement of hydrogen ion concentration
____	8. Ketosus	________	H. Narrow strip of plastic used in urinalysis to detect a variety of substances and values
____	9. Crystals	________	I. Insoluble matter that settles to the bottom of a liquid; material examined in the urinalysis microscopic examination
____	10. Midstream	________	J. Opaque; lack of clarity
____	11. Supernatant	________	K. Condition that occurs when the net rate at which the body produces acids or bases is equal to the net rate at which acids or bases are excreted
____	12. Regent test strip	________	L. Tiny structures usually formed by deposits of protein (or other substances) within the walls of renal tubules

	Column A	Correct Spelling	Column B
____	13. Urea	____________	M. Urine sample collected in the middle of the flow of urine
____	14. Turbid	____________	N. Principal end product of protein metabolism
____	15. Acid–base balance	____________	O. Found in normal urine sediment, these structures generally have no particular significance; the presence of a few should be noted because they may indicate disease states
____	16. UTI	____________	P. Ratio of weight of a given volume of a substance to the weight of the same volume of distilled water at the same temperature; test often performed during the urinalysis physical examination (can also appear on the reagent strip)

Terms

Fill in the proper terms relating to urinalysis.

______________ 1. Orange-yellow pigment that forms from the breakdown of hemoglobin in red blood cells; usually travels in the bloodstream to the liver, where it is converted to a water-soluble form and excreted into the bile

______________ 2. Abnormal presence of blood in urine, symptomatic of many disorders of the genitourinary system and renal diseases

______________ 3. Colorless compound produced in the intestines after the breakdown by bacteria of bilirubin

______________ 4. Accumulation of ketones in the body, occurring primarily as a complication of diabetes mellitus; if left untreated, it could cause coma

______________ 5. Pattern based on 24-hour cycle that emphasizes the repetition of certain physiologic phenomena such as eating and sleeping

______________ 6. Waste product formed in muscle that is excreted by the kidneys; increased in blood and urine when kidney function is abnormal

______________ 7. Instrument that measures the refractive index of a substance or solution; used in the urinalysis chemical examination to measure the urine specimen's specific gravity

______________ 8. Urine that appears to be above the sediment when centrifuged; poured off before sediment is examined in the urinalysis microscopic examination

LEARNING REVIEW

Short Answer

1. After passing through a healthy kidney, urine composition is approximately __% water and __% percent dissolved substances, which generally come from dietary intake or metabolic waste products.

2. Identify each substance below as a normal (N) or an abnormal (AB) substance found in urine.

Urobilinogen ___

Potassium ___

Uric acid ___

White blood cells ___

Fat ___

Protein ___

Blood ___

Creatinine ___

Chloride ___

3. When handling urine specimens, Standard Precautions must be followed to ensure that proper infection control standards are observed. In the space provided below, list three precautions used when handling urine specimens.

____

____

____

____

4. List seven regulations of the Clinical Laboratory Improvement Act (CLIA) that apply to the clinical medical assistant performing urine testing.

____

____

____

____

____

____

5. What are the four steps in a physical examination of a urine specimen?

____

____

____

____

6. What does the specific gravity of urine indicate?

____

____

____

____

7. How should reagent test strips be handled and stored?

____

____

____

____

8. Casts are formed when protein accumulates and precipitates in the kidney tubules and are then washed into the urine. Identify each cast below and draw an example in the space provided.

Description	Cast Name	Drawing
These casts contain remnants of disintegrated cells that have a fine or coarse appearance.	________	
These casts may contain epithelial cells, red blood cells, or white blood cells.	________	
These casts can be seen in normal urine but increase with any kidney disease. They can also be seen as a result of fever, emotional stress, or strenuous exercise. These casts are nearly transparent and can be difficult to see under the microscope without some light adjustment.	________	

9. In the space below, draw an example of each type of sediment as seen under a microscope.

Drawing	Sediment
	Sperm, cotton fibers, and starch granules
	Yeast
	Bacteria

Matching

Microscopic examination of urine sediment is a valuable diagnostic tool for providers. Match each type of sediment to the statement that best describes it.

A. White blood cells

B. Yeast

C. Squamous epithelial cells

D. Renal tubular epithelial cells

E. Bacteria

F. Artifacts

G. Red blood cells

H. Parasites

I. Sperm

_____ Hair, fiber, powder, and oil are common examples.

_____ These skin cells are not medically significant and are sloughed off into the urine.

_____ *Trichomonas vaginalis* is the type most frequently seen in urine.

_____ Can appear as tiny round or rod-shaped objects, often seem to be shaking or vibrating.

_____ These cells appear as pale, light-refractive disks; they are counted in a microscopic field and reported as cells per high-power field (HPF).

_____ These cells are larger than red blood cells, have a visible nucleus, and may appear granular.

_____ These cells are reported when seen in male and female urine.

_____ *Candida albicans* is the most common example.

_____ These cells can indicate kidney disease if present in large numbers and are easily confused with other surface cells.

CERTIFICATION REVIEW

These questions are designed to mimic the certification examination. Select the best response.

1. What is the filtering unit of the kidney called?
   a. Meatus
   b. Glomerulus
   c. Ureter
   d. Urethra

2. What is the common medication used to treat bladder infections and turns the urine bright orange?
   a. Pyridium
   b. Zestoretic
   c. Propranolol
   d. Neurontin
   e. Omeprozole

3. What smell will the urine of a patient with diabetes who has ketoacidosis have?
   a. Musty
   b. Sour
   c. Putrid
   d. Sweet

4. What is the curvature that appears in a liquid's upper surface when placed in a container?
   a. Specific gravity
   b. Urobilinogen
   c. Meniscus
   d. Buffy coat
   e. Billirubin

5. What type of cast seen in urine sediment can be a result of fever, emotional stress, or strenuous exercise?
   a. Hyaline
   b. Granular
   c. Waxy
   d. Cellular

6. Which part of the urinalysis is to be performed by the provider?
   a. Chemical examination
   b. Physical examination
   c. Specific gravity
   d. Microscopic examination
   e. Quantitative test

7. What forms in urine whenever the body uses fat/fatty acids for energy rather than carbohydrates/sugars?
   a. Diabetes
   b. Lipolysis
   c. Cystitis
   d. Ketones
   e. Both a and b

8. If the patient brings a urine sample in a household container from home for a complete urinalysis, what should you do?
   a. Accept it this time, but for subsequent tests, you will give them a proper container
   b. Provide the patient with an appropriate container and ask for a fresh sample
   c. Carefully and politely explain to the patient why you require a freshly voided specimen in a sterile container
   d. Check the seal and if intact, perform the UA
   e. Both b and c

9. What is the most common urine specimen type in the provider's office laboratory (POL)?
   a. Sterile specimen
   b. Timed specimen
   c. Random specimen
   d. Catheterized specimen

10. Neutral pH is measured at 7. If a specimen has a pH of 5.3, what concentration is it?
   a. Alkaline
   b. Acidic
   c. Base
   d. Low-level concentration
   e. None of the above

LEARNING APPLICATION

Critical Thinking

1. What is the importance of proper urine collection?

____

____

____

____

2. When is a urine preservative necessary?

3. What would give a urine sample a cloudy appearance?

4. Why do you suppose we test for sugar in urine but not salt/sodium?

5. If a medical assistant is color blind, does that mean he or she cannot perform the chemical testing of urine? What (if any) accommodations can be made for him or her?

Case Studies

CASE STUDY 1

At Inner City Health Care, Gwen Carr, CMA (AAMA), gives patient Wendy Janus written directions for a 24-hour urine collection to be performed at home, but Wendy misplaces them. Gwen must now give directions to Wendy over the telephone.

CASE STUDY REVIEW QUESTIONS

1. What directions should be given to the patient to correctly perform the urine collection?

2. What communication techniques should Gwen use to make sure the patient understands the collection procedures? What other potential alternatives for communicating the information, besides the telephone, are available?

CASE STUDY 2

Nancy McFarland, RMA (AMT), is asked to tell a male adolescent patient the proper procedure for a clean-catch specimen. The 15-year-old boy is visibly embarrassed and will not hold eye contact with Nancy as she relates the instructions for collection.

CASE STUDY REVIEW QUESTIONS

1. What instructions are relevant for a clean-catch specimen for this patient?

2. What communication techniques should Nancy use when working with this patient?

CASE STUDY 3

Your patient comes in with complaints of severe lower abdominal pain, burning, frequency, and blood in her urine. When you ask her for a urine sample for testing, she is able to give only about 6 mL because of the frequency of her urination.

1. Will you be able to perform any testing on the 6-mL specimen?

Hands-on Activities

1. One of the most important steps in the collection of urine specimens is to correctly identify the specimen through proper labeling. Make up your own identification number, using Dr. Mark King as your provider, and write out complete labeling information for a specimen of urine below, using your own name for the patient's name.

2. What is the proper procedure for testing an unlabeled or incorrectly labeled specimen?

ATTRIBUTES OF PROFESSIONALISM

Examination of urine (urinalysis) has been performed for centuries by medical practitioners as a diagnostic tool for many diseases. Urinalysis refers to the study of urine as an aid in diagnosis or to follow the course of disease. The urine examination is a routine part of most physical examinations. Practice, experience, and attention to detail are the most important tools in achieving quality results. Think about what you have learned in this chapter and, in your journal, consider your personal experiences and the Attributes of Professionalism as you answer the following questions.

1. Have you ever had a urinalysis performed?

2. If you have had a urinalysis performed, were you given proper instructions for a urinalysis? If not, why do you think you were not instructed properly? If you were, did you understand clearly what you were to do?

3. Were instructions clearly written and posted in the restroom at a location that was readable during the collection?

4. Do you think that good patient preparation and instructions influence the result of the test performed? In what way?

5. Now that you know the importance of proper patient instruction, how will your experience and training influence your work as a medical assistant in other areas of patient education?

Name ______________________ Date ________ Score ________

CHAPTER 42

Basic Microbiology

VOCABULARY BUILDER

Misspelled Words

Find the words in Column A that are misspelled; circle them, and then correctly spell them in the spaces provided. Then match each vocabulary term below with the correct definition in Column B.

	Column A	Correct Spelling	Column B
____	1. Erobic	____________	A. The science and study of fungi
____	2. Arasols	____________	B. The act of coughing up material from the air passages
____	3. Genus	____________	C. Infection acquired in a hospital
____	4. Anerobic	____________	D. Bacteria that are suspended in a liquid since living organisms will not live long in dry conditions, especially near the heat of the microscope light
____	5. Mycology	____________	E. Bacteria encapsulated in protein, providing protection from antibiotic penetration and white blood cell attack
____	6. Inccubate	____________	F. Living only in the presence of oxygen
____	7. Gram stain	____________	G. The naming of
____	8. Inoculate	____________	H. Living only in the absence of oxygen
____	9. Nosacomal	____________	I. To grow, as in a culture
____	10. Expectorate	____________	J. To place colonies of microorganisms onto nutrient media
____	11. Normal floura	____________	K. Applied to bacteria to differentiate two basic groups, either positive or negative
____	12. Morphology	____________	L. Natural bacteria
____	13. Nomenclature	____________	M. The science of structure and form without regard to function
____	14. Spores	____________	N. The classification between family and species
____	15. Wet mount	____________	O. Airborne particles that can be released into the air when culturing

LEARNING REVIEW

Fill in the Blanks

1. Infections from parasites have increased as more people travel and public awareness of the symptoms grows. The most common parasitic infections seen in the laboratory are ________________, the causative organism of pinworm infection, and ________________, a parasite that infects the urogenital tracts of men and women.

2. Tests for parasites are usually performed on body fluids and excretions such as ________________, ________________, and ________________.

3. Labeling specimens sent for testing with ________________, ________________, and ________________ collected is important, as well as noting if the patient has been ________________ to a specific place and what diagnosis the provider suspects.

4. ________________________ should be worn when working with specimens. Assuming that all specimens are infectious is an important element of following ________________ for infection control.

5. The practice of proper aseptic ________________ several times a day, including after glove removal, is essential and should become a ________________.

Short Answer

1. Specimen containers will arrive at the laboratory inside biohazard plastic transport bags to avoid danger to laboratory personnel. What precautions are taken before opening the bags?

2. A laboratory's success in finding and identifying a pathogenic organism in a sample depends on multiple factors. Name eight.

3. The medical assistant in a provider's office will most likely frequently assist in the care and treatment of patients with sore throats.

   A. Why is it necessary to rapidly identify the cause?

   B. What test would be used to determine the cause of a sore throat?

C. What five rules should be followed when conducting the test referenced in the previous question?

____

____

____

____

4. Label the parts of the cell, referring to the following image. Then check *Sometimes* for the parts that are sometimes present and *Always* for the parts that are always present.

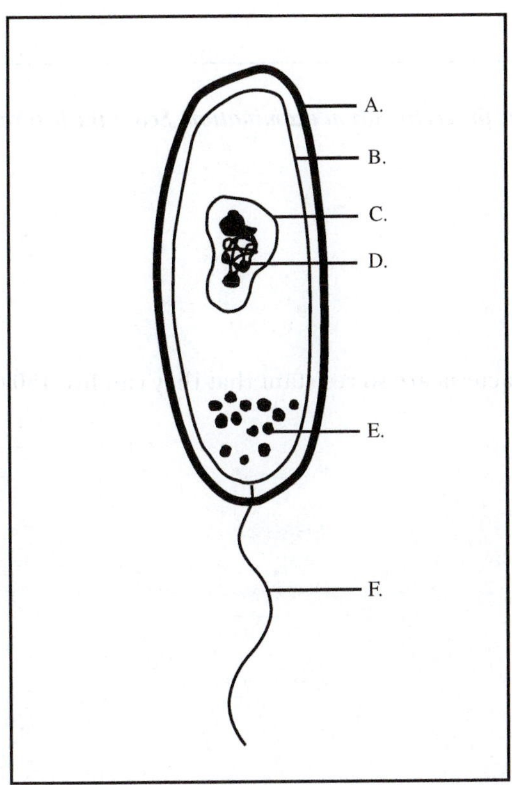

Label	Sometimes	Always
A. ____________	______	______
B. ____________	______	______
C. ____________	______	______
D. ____________	______	______
E. ____________	______	______
F. ____________	______	______

5. Describe the process of sensitivity testing and explain why it is an important tool.

____

____

____

____

____

CERTIFICATION REVIEW

These questions are designed to mimic the certification examination. Select the best response.

1. Which organism causes boils?
   a. *Salmonella*
   b. *Staphylococcus*
   c. *Shigella*
   d. Protista

2. What type/characteristics of bacteria are so resistant that they can live 150,000 years?
   a. Flagella
   b. Cell walls
   c. Nuclei
   d. Spores
   e. None of the above

3. What is septicemia?
   a. Blood infection
   b. Throat infection
   c. Urinary tract infection
   d. Respiratory infection

4. What shape best describes bacilli?
   a. Rod
   b. Round
   c. Spiral
   d. Clusters
   e. Motile

5. What color does gram-negative bacteria stain?
   a. Purple
   b. Pink
   c. Red
   d. Green

6. CSF cultures must be tested as what type of specimen?
   a. Timed specimen
   b. ASAP specimen
   c. STAT specimen
   d. Random specimen
   e. POL-tested specimen

7. Bacteria that remain purple in the staining process are known as what?
   a. Gram positive
   b. Gram negative
   c. Acid-fast
   d. None of the above

8. What organism requires CO_2?
   a. *Streptococcus*
   b. *Clostridium*
   c. *Salmonella*
   d. *Neisseria gonorrhoeae*
   e. *Escherichia coli*

9. Most fecal specimens being tested for ova or parasitic infestations are stored at what temperature?
   a. Between room temperature and body temperature
   b. Body temperature (98.6°F)
   c. Refrigerated
   d. Frozen

10. *Candida* species present a particular problem in the health care setting, where they can cause serious nosocomial infections. What does nosocomial refer to?
    a. Infections caused by hospital and medical procedures
    b. Infections caused by sexual contact
    c. Infections caused by contact with a person infected with HIV
    d. *Neisseria gonorrhoeae*
    e. Both b and d

LEARNING APPLICATION

Critical Thinking

1. What is liquid suspension and what special situations make this a better aid to bacterial identification than staining?

   ____

   ____

2. Define aerosols and explain how protection is provided when the medical assistant is working with an aerosol.

3. Identify one potential pathogen and list the specimen source, media for culture, microscopic appearance, and disease it causes.

4. Explain why pinworm specimens are collected at a specific time of the day.

Case Studies

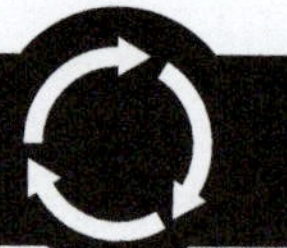

CASE STUDY 1

Dr. Winston Lewis has ordered a series of three sputum cultures for Herb Fowler, who has had a productive cough for several months along with extreme fatigue. Joe Guerrero, CMA (AAMA), is assigned to obtain the cultures. When the cultures are obtained from Mr. Fowler, Joe brings them to the POL for culturing.

CASE STUDY REVIEW QUESTIONS

1. What is the procedure for obtaining a sputum specimen?

Research Activity

Make a list of all the things that are done to keep your food and other aspects of your environment free of pathogens, including water purification, food processing, homogenization, use of antibacterial soap and cleansers, immunizations, and any other process you can think of.

1. After each item on the list, place a check mark by those that are available only to certain populations but not to underdeveloped countries and areas.

2. Discuss with your classmates which of the things on your lists could be implemented fairly simply and inexpensively in underdeveloped countries. List those items below.

3. Reorganize each list, starting with the easiest to implement and moving toward the most expensive/difficult.

4. List other items or processes that would need to be done to implement each item on your list.

ATTRIBUTES OF PROFESSIONALISM

After completing this chapter, describe how you feel about working with patients who have infections that are possibly communicable. What, if anything, concerns you? What resources can help you address your concerns? Describe how you will apply the Attributes of Professionalism when working with patients that may have a communicable disease. Cite specific examples.

Name ______________________ Date __________ Score __________

CHAPTER 43

Specialty Laboratory Tests

VOCABULARY BUILDER

Misspelled Words

Find the words listed below that are misspelled; circle them, and correctly spell them in the spaces provided. Then insert the vocabulary terms into the sentences that follow. Not all terms will be used.

ABO blood group	Guthrie screening test	Mantous test
billirubin	high-density lipoprotein	phenylketonuria (PKU)
blood urea nitrogin	human chorionic gonadotropin (hCG)	purified protein derivative (PPD)
chalesterol	low-density lipoprotein	Rh factor
enduration		tryglicerides

______________________ ______________________ ______________________

______________________ ______________________ ______________________

1. Although PPD is used to test for tuberculosis, the name of the test is the ______________________ test after the physician who developed it.

2. To evaluate a newborn for PKU, Thomas Myers, CCMA (NHA), uses the ______________________ to evaluate the baby's blood.

3. When Mary O'Keefe's enzyme immunoassay test is positive, Gwen Carr, CMA (AAMA), assumes that this positive reaction indicates a normal pregnancy. However, detection of hCG, ______________________, can also indicate abnormal conditions such as an ectopic pregnancy.

4. High levels of ______________________, "bad" cholesterol, are associated with an increased risk for coronary artery disease. Cholesterol bound to ______________________, "good" cholesterol, is transported to the liver, where it is excreted in the form of bile.

5. Serum ______________________ concentration will increase moderately after a patient ingests a meal containing fat, and the concentration will peak 4 to 5 hours later.

6. Nora Fowler was born with ____________________, an inherited condition in which a baby does not have the enzyme that metabolizes the phenylalanine amino acid into tyrosine amino acid properly.

7. When renal disease is suspected, a physician will order, as one of several tests, a ____________________ test, which measures the concentration of urea in the blood.

8. Patients exhibiting a positive or questionable ____________________ reaction should have a chest X-ray study to examine for tubercules, and a sputum sample should be stained to search for acid-fast rods. The presence of tubercules and ____________________ rods confirms active tuberculosis.

9. Two categories of blood typing are for the ____________________ and the ____________________.

LEARNING REVIEW

Short Answer

1. Name three reasons for performing a semen analysis on a male patient.

____

____

____

2. When a semen analysis is performed as part of a fertility workup, seminal fluid is analyzed to determine what factors? Name at least four.

____

____

____

3. Name the four blood group categories.

____

____

____

4. Fill in the missing information in the chart below.

Blood Group/Type	Antigen on RBC	Serum Antibodies
AB	________	________
________	B	________
________	________	Anti-B

5. Explain the difference between saturated, monounsaturated, and polyunsaturated fats and give an example of each.

____

____

____

6. What are some ways that quality control can be maintained when performing waived-category tests in the POL?

____

____

____

7. List three specialty tests from the CLIA-waived category that might be performed in the POL and what type of specimen is needed for each.

____

____

Fill in the Blanks

Fill in the blanks with the correct term.

1. The Rh type of most North Americans is ________________.
2. Glucose is the principal carbohydrate found circulating in the ________________.
3. Excess glucose is converted into ________________ for short-term storage in the liver and muscle cells.
4. After consumption of the glucose test solution, the blood glucose level of patients without ________________ usually peaks within 30 to 60 minutes, leading to a level of 160 to 180 mg/dL, and then returns to the fasting level after 2 to 3 hours.
5. To determine whether patients with diabetes are consistently adhering to their diets, providers can administer the ________________________________.

CERTIFICATION REVIEW

These questions are designed to mimic the certification examination. Select the best response.

1. Blood types are based on the presence or absence of what on the surface of red blood cells (RBCs)?
   a. Antigens
   b. Antibodies
   c. Immunoglobulins
   d. Electrolytes
2. What is a potentially life-threatening situation during incompatible blood transfusion called?
   a. Epstein-Barr
   b. Intravascular hemolysis
   c. Hydatidiform mole
   d. Phenylketonuria
   e. None of the above
3. Men with oligospermia should be evaluated for which type of disorder?
   a. Pancreatic
   b. Hepatic
   c. Thyroid
   d. Renal
4. Which of the following reflects a negative reaction to a Mantoux test?
   a. 10-mm induration or more
   b. 5- to 9-mm induration
   c. 12- to 15-mm induration
   d. Less than 5-mm induration or without induration
   e. Greater than 15-mm induration

5. What does postprandial refer to?
   a. After eating
   b. After medication
   c. After sleeping
   d. After urinating

6. Insulin is secreted by which organ?
   a. Liver
   b. Spleen
   c. Kidney
   d. Pancreas
   e. Gallbladder

7. When performing the Mantoux test, what size needle would you choose?
   a. 24 gauge, ½ inch
   b. 25 gauge, ⅜ inch
   c. 26 to 27 gauge, ½ inch
   d. 28 to 30 gauge, ⅜ inch

8. Which of the following factors can alter the results of semen analysis?
   a. Eating foods containing garlic
   b. Smoking cigarettes
   c. Riding a bicycle on the day of the analysis
   d. Drinking milk
   e. Drinking sugary beverages

9. Which of the following is not a symptom of infectious mononucleosis?
   a. Swollen extremities
   b. Swollen glands
   c. Swollen spleen
   d. Swollen lymph nodes

10. Which of the following factors may influence the Guthrie test?
   a. Experiencing feeding problems such as vomiting
   b. Failing to ingest sufficient phenylalanine
   c. Taking aspirin
   d. Taking antibiotics
   e. All of the above

LEARNING APPLICATION

1. What factors may alter the results of a blood glucose measurement?

____

____

2. How can you distinguish between patients who have diabetes and do not have diabetes based on results of the 2-hour postprandial glucose evaluation?

3. What is the function of triglycerides in the body?

4. What is the source of urea in the blood?

Case Studies

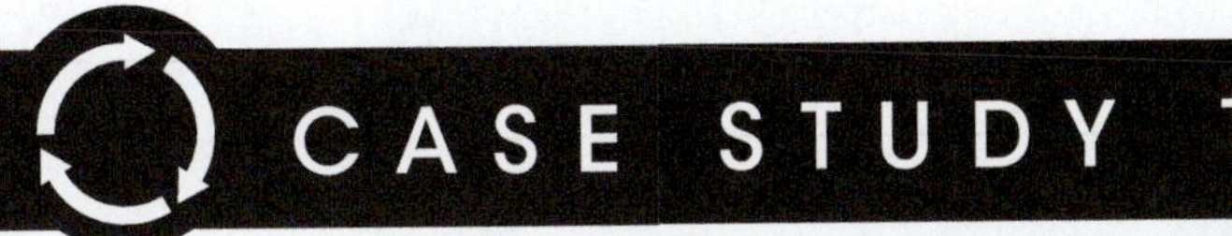

Mary Alexander is an established patient of Dr. Lewis's at Inner City Health Care. Mary, 32 years old, is about 10 pounds overweight for her height. Mary was diagnosed with type 1 insulin-dependent diabetes mellitus when she was a child. Dr. Lewis's treatment plan includes administration of 30 units of U-100 NPH insulin by injection every day. Dr. Lewis knows that Mary has trouble complying with the dietary restrictions included in her treatment plan and with observing regular mealtimes. Every now and then, the stress of the diet wears Mary down and she begins to eat whatever she likes, whenever she feels like it. As a safeguard, Dr. Lewis asks Mary to report her average glucose levels to Joe Guerrero, CMA (AAMA), twice monthly. At her next regular follow-up examination with Dr. Lewis, the physician orders a glycosated hemoglobin determination (HbA1c) and discovers that Mary has not been complying with her diet and has been reporting inaccurate glucose levels to the physician's office, hoping Dr. Lewis would not find out.

CASE STUDY REVIEW QUESTIONS

1. How is Dr. Lewis able to tell from the glycosylated hemoglobin determination (HbA1c) that Mary is not adhering to her diet?

2. What is glycosated hemoglobin?

CASE STUDY 2

Your patient, an immigrant from Vietnam, is entering a medical assisting program and needs to be tested for TB. She is concerned because she received the BCG vaccination in Vietnam and was told by her friends that she will always react to the PPD test even if she doesn't have TB because of the BCG vaccination. She has many questions.

CASE STUDY REVIEW QUESTIONS

1. Why does she need to have the Mantoux test if she will always react because of the BCG?

___

___

___

2. Will she always react to the PPD?

___

___

3. Will she still need to have a chest X-ray study?

___

4. Does she have TB?

___

5. Is she protected from getting TB by the BCG vaccination?

___

6. Does she need treatment?

___

___

Research Activities

1. Do an Internet investigation to see if your state requires PKU testing on newborns.
   a. If not, why do you think it is not required? Is the test recommended? How much does it cost? Do you think the law should be changed? Why or why not?
   b. If your state does require it, are parents allowed to refuse? Why would a parent refuse?
   c. Role-play with another student: How would you react if a parent refused?
2. Look at Table 43-4 (Values for Cholesterol, HDL, LDL, and Triglycerides) in your textbook. What are the normal ranges of each for your gender?

___

___

ATTRIBUTES OF PROFESSIONALISM

This chapter covers a variety of specialty laboratory tests. Select one or two of the tests covered in the text, and write in your journal how you would apply the Attributes of Professionalism in performing these tests and communicating with the patient regarding the tests and results. Cite specific examples of professionalism required.

Name ______________________ Date __________ Score __________

CHAPTER 44

The Medical Assistant as Clinic Manager

VOCABULARY BUILDER

Misspelled Words

Find the words listed below that are misspelled; circle them, and correctly spell them in the spaces provided. Then insert the correct vocabulary terms in the sentences that follow.

agenda	"going bare"	procedure manual
ancilliary services	itinerary	professional liability insurance
benchmark	marketting	risk managment
benifit	minutes	teamwork
bond	negligance	work statement
embezzel	practicum	

______________________ ______________________ ______________________

______________________ ______________________ ______________________

1. ______________________ Professional occupational companies hired to complete a specific job such as janitorial services, laundry, or disposal of hazardous materials

2. ______________________ Refers to the situation of a provider who does not carry insurance to protect the provider's assets in the event of a liability claim

3. ______________________ A comparison between different organizations relative to how they accomplish tasks, remunerate employees, and so on

4. ______________________ Designed to protect assets in the event a liability claim is filed and awarded

5. ______________________ A written record of topics discussed and actions taken during meeting sessions

6. ______________________ Provides a concise description of the work you plan to accomplish

7. ______________ A binding agreement with an employee ensuring recovery of financial loss should funds be stolen or embezzled

8. ______________ A printed list of topics to be discussed during a meeting

9. ______________ The process by which the provider of services makes the consumer aware of the scope and quality of those services; examples include public relations, brochures, patient education seminars, and newsletters

10. ______________ Involves persons synergistically working together

11. ______________ A transitional stage providing an opportunity to apply theory learned in the classroom to a health care setting through practical, hands-on experience

12. ______________ Remuneration that is in addition to a salary

13. ______________ To appropriate fraudulently for one's own use

14. ______________ Involves the identification, analysis, and treatment of risks within the medical clinic

15. ______________ Occurs when one performs an act that a reasonable and prudent provider would not perform or fails to perform an act that a reasonable and prudent provider would perform

16. ______________ Provides detailed information relative to the performance of tasks within the facility in which one is employed

17. ______________ A detailed plan for a proposed trip

LEARNING REVIEW

Short Answer

1. The manager of a medical clinic or ambulatory care facility can have many varied responsibilities based on individual facility needs. What are six duties that are the responsibility of the clinic manager in a health care setting?

____

____

____

____

____

____

____

____

____

2. What are five attributes needed to excel as a manager/leader in any clinic setting?

____

____

3. List four suggestions that are proven means of managing your time, whether in management or as a salaried employee.

____

4. What is the difference between authoritarian and participatory management styles?

5. What does "management by walking around" mean, and why would it be useful in a medical clinic setting?

6. The table below outlines some of the common risks for medical clinics, as well as risk control measures for each risk. Fill in any missing information.

Risk	Risk Control Measures
	Train various employees to assume other duties and perform them when an employee is ill, on vacation, etc.
Failure of a supplier or contractor	
	Have protocols in place for handling this situation and make patients aware of the protocols; notify patients immediately if confidential information is disclosed and work with them toward resolution
Computer failure	
	Continually review safety procedures, conduct safety surveys, always carry liability insurance, complete an incident report to signal the risk manager to implement existing protocols to minimize risk

7. Define harassment in the workplace.

8. List the steps and precautions that a manager should take if he or she is made aware of harassment in the medical clinic.

9. Why do some employers put new employees on probation? What is the usual length of an employee's probationary period?

Ordering Activity

All administrative and clinical supplies and equipment in the facility must be inventoried. The following tasks are performed when new supplies and/or equipment are received. Put the tasks in the correct order, from 1 to 5.

_____ A. Unpack each item, checking against the packing slip

_____ B. Write the date the shipment was received and who verified it

_____ C. Stock each item and store appropriately

_____ D. Verify that no items have been substituted or back-ordered

_____ E. Find the packing slip listing the items ordered

Matching

Most marketing tools used in a medical environment provide educational and clinic services information to patients, potential patients, and the local community. Match the following marketing tools with their potential use in the ambulatory care facility setting.

A. Seminars
B. Brochures
C. Newsletters
D. Press releases
E. Special events
F. Social media

_______ 1. These are a way to announce clinic expansions, new equipment, providers joining the practice, or add-on services and affiliations with area facilities.

_______ 2. These typically address two areas—patient education and clinic services—and present a professional image of the ambulatory care setting. This information must always be updated. These describe the clinic, HIPAA policies, insurance and payment information, provider profiles, and scope of services for the patient.

_______ 3. These provide an effective way to join with other community organizations to promote wellness.

_______ 4. These can educate patients and provide goodwill in the community. All facility staff can work as a team to organize these.

_______ 5. This is an optimal way to offer health-related articles, including clinic updates such as policy changes, staff introductions, and insurance information. Typically released biannually or quarterly, these can be made available in the waiting room.

_______ 6. Digital forms of communication such as Facebook, Twitter, and blogging are not only necessary marketing tools but excellent ways to keep information updated and available to patients and visitors seeking information.

CERTIFICATION REVIEW

These questions are designed to mimic the certification examination. Select the best response.

1. Social media is a good way to project what information about a clinic?
   a. Technical expertise
   b. Educational level
   c. Personality
   d. Salary
2. Why do most conflicts occur between employees and supervisors or providers?
   a. Unreasonable expectations
   b. Poor communication
   c. Misunderstandings
   d. Unfair or inappropriately given criticism
   e. All of the above
3. With which management style does each staff member feel that he or she can or has made a contribution, increasing the sense of value within the team?
   a. Participatory
   b. Authoritarian
   c. Compromising
   d. Teaching and coaching
   e. All of the above

4. Checking for any frayed electrical cords, loose connections, or safety issues such as tripping hazards is known as practicing what?
   a. SDS functions
   b. Physical plant analysis
   c. Risk management principles
   d. Physical plant inventory
   e. Equipment and supply maintenance

5. What steps should the clinic manager take to determine wages and salaries for employees with comparable skills?
   a. Network
   b. Interview employees
   c. Search the largest city in the state for minimum-wage law
   d. Defer to the provider only for wage determination

6. What is a rule that defines almost all of a manager's ethical qualities?
   a. Murphy's law
   b. The rule of nines
   c. The golden rule
   d. The ethics of medicine rule
   e. None of the above

7. What management style/technique promotes face-to-face conversations, obtaining feedback, and listening to staff ideas or comments?
   a. Walking around
   b. Participatory
   c. Risk
   d. Authoritarian

8. What is the most significant task of the team leader or clinic manager?
   a. Getting the team members to understand and support the specifics of the problem they are asked to solve
   b. Enabling the team to develop their own work statement through which they will assume ownership of the goals and objectives
   c. Establishing a timetable for achieving results and identifying the standards that must be maintained
   d. All of the above
   e. Only a and c

9. Which of the following is associated with being a leader?
   a. Organizing and allocating talent and resources
   b. Controlling and solving problems, with the ability to adapt to changes seamlessly
   c. Consistently achieving goals and targets
   d. Being an inspiring and motivating influence, able to mentor and direct in ways that keep the team moving forward

10. If malpractice litigation should occur, what is the best protocol to follow?
    a. Be honest with the patients and insurance carriers
    b. Let the HR person handle the situation
    c. Notify the provider
    d. Do not get involved
    e. Correct the patient chart by deleting information that is harmful to the provider/practice

LEARNING APPLICATION

Critical Thinking

1. How would you, as the clinic manager, handle someone who is spreading an awful rumor about another employee in the clinic?

2. How can the clinic manager promote open and honest communication?

3. The student practicum can be a stressful time for the extern. As the clinic manager, how can you help the extern feel more at ease the first day of "work"?

4. Describe how a procedure manual for a single-provider practice would differ from a procedure manual for a multiprovider practice.

5. Describe how a procedure manual could become outdated, and the steps for revision.

Case Studies

CASE STUDY 1

Clinic manager Marilyn Johnson, CMA (AAMA), is responsible for the preparation and distribution of payroll checks at Inner City Health Care. Because the group practice is in the process of upgrading the computer system to accommodate a recent influx of new patients, Marilyn is temporarily preparing the payroll using the manual write-it-once bookkeeping system. She is careful to consult payroll records for each employee, which include the employee's name, address, telephone number, and Social Security number; number of exemptions claimed on the W-4 form; gross salary; deductions withheld for all taxes, including Social Security, federal, state, and local; deductions withheld for health insurance and disability insurance; and date of employment.

CASE STUDY REVIEW QUESTIONS

1. As Marilyn writes out the payroll check for Gwen Carr, CMA (AAMA), what information should be included on the paycheck stub?

2. What must the provider's clinic have to process payroll?

3. What responsibility does the clinic manager have with regard to the confidentiality of payroll records? How might employees' rights to privacy be maintained?

ATTRIBUTES OF PROFESSIONALISM

Put yourself in the place of the clinic manager. Good managers are leaders, providing their co-workers with vision, guidance, and a feeling of ownership in the process. They do these things without threats, usually through the power of their personal charisma. It is also important that managers clearly convey their expectations to their employees. Possibly nothing leads to ill feelings between a manager and an employee more than failure to set clear expectations. Furthermore, a lack of expectations stifles career growth and organizational vitality. Good leaders need to blend many admirable personality traits of leadership to be successful and still control the resources entrusted to them.

With the Attributes of Professionalism in mind, do an honest self-assessment and ask yourself, "Would I want to be a clinic manager?" "What kind of clinic manager would I be?" Detail in your journal how you reached your conclusion and what type of management style you think you are the most comfortable with. What skills come naturally to you and what skills will you have to work on the most?

Name____________________ Date________ Score________

CHAPTER **45**

The Medical Assistant as Human Resources Manager

VOCABULARY BUILDER

Misspelled Words

Find the words listed below that are misspelled; circle them, and correctly spell them in the spaces provided. Then, insert the correct vocabulary terms into the following sentences.

Boomer genneration	involuntary dismisal	overtime
exit interveiw	letter of resignation	probation
________________	________________	________________
________________	________________	________________

1. Because of an unexpected staffing shortfall, Nancy McFarland, RMA (AMT), has volunteered to work ________________ this week. She will receive 1.5 times the regular rate of pay for hours above her regular 40-hour week.

2. An ________________ has been scheduled for administrative/clinical medical assistant Liz Corbin, CMA (AAMA), before she leaves the clinic to continue her education. This session will give Liz an opportunity to provide her positive and negative opinions of the position and the facility.

3. The violation of clinic policies at Inner City Health Care led to the ________________ of one of the part-time employees.

4. Liz Corbin, CMA (AAMA), submitted a ________________ to her current employer when she decided to leave her present position to return to school to pursue an advanced degree.

5. Clinic manager Marilyn Johnson, CMA (AAMA), will inform all of the job applicants that they will be on ________________ for their first 30 to 60 days in the position. During this period, the employee and supervisory personnel can determine if the environment and the position are satisfactory for the employee.

6. The ________________, born from 1955 to 1965, may still struggle with the vast advancement of technology in all aspects of their work.

LEARNING REVIEW

Short Answer

1. The manual that identifies clear guidelines and directions required of all employees is known as the policy manual. What are four topics identified in this chapter that would be included in a policy manual, regardless of the size of the practice?

2. Clinic manager Marilyn Johnson, CMA (AAMA), has the responsibility of dismissing an employee for a serious violation of clinic policies. From the list below, select key points to keep in mind when dismissal is necessary by circling the letters of the statements that apply.
   a. Pack the employee's belongings from his or her desk
   b. Verbal and written warnings must be given to the employee and are to be well documented
   c. Allow as much time as possible to interview the employee for the dismissal
   d. Be flexible in listening to the employee's side of the story, including any impact on his or her family
   e. Explain terms of dismissal (keys, clearing out area, final paperwork)
   f. To be fair, listen to the employee's emotions
   g. If a clinic manager expects any serious difficulties with an employee during an immediate dismissal, the HR director or another person appointed to assist should be present when the employee is notified

3. Compare and contrast voluntary and involuntary separation.

4. The job description must have enough information to provide both the supervisor and the employee with a clear outline of what the job entails. Name four items that must be included in a job description.

5. Name six items that should be included on any interview worksheet.

CERTIFICATION REVIEW

These questions are designed to mimic the certification examination. Select the best response.

1. Although salary discussions are typically left to the second interview, which of the following would be an appropriate question from the manager during a first interview?
   a. Are you aware of how much the position pays?
   b. Are you expecting more than the minimum wage?
   c. What salary are you expecting?
   d. Are you aware the salary for this position has not been determined?

2. How are questions regarding substance abuse, arrest records, and medical history during an interview viewed?
   a. Appropriate
   b. Inappropriate
   c. Illegal
   d. Legal and appropriate
   e. Both b and c

3. Title VII of the Civil Rights Act addresses which of the following topics?
   a. Overtime pay
   b. Discrimination based on race, age, and sex
   c. Hiring and firing practices
   d. Sexual harassment

4. When a candidate accepts a position, the HR manager should write what type of letter that clearly spells out details of the discussion and outlines the specifics of the position?
   a. Confirmation letter
   b. Congratulatory letter
   c. Recommendation letter
   d. Reference letter
   e. Letter of understanding

5. A person with AIDS who satisfies the necessary skills for a position and has the experience and education required will be protected from discrimination by which of the following agencies/acts?
   a. OSHA
   b. CLIA
   c. AAMA
   d. ADA

6. How often should a job description be reviewed and updated?
   a. Every 2 years
   b. Every 90 days
   c. Every year
   d. Every 5 years
   e. Only when a position is vacated

7. When does voluntary separation usually occur?
   a. When advancing to another position
   b. When there is a violation of clinic policies
   c. When the employee is relocating
   d. Both a and c

8. How is a new employee verified as being authorized to work?
   a. Ask for verbal clarification
   b. Have the candidate complete an I-9 form
   c. Have the candidate provide a notarized statement
   d. Have the candidate fill out an attestation form
   e. Have the candidate provide a valid passport

9. Which of the following documents is not included in the employee personnel file?
   a. Application
   b. Formal review
   c. Name, address, telephone number, and Social Security number
   d. Employee handbook

10. What act was established to prevent injuries and illnesses resulting from unsafe and unhealthy working conditions?
    a. Americans with Disabilities Act
    b. Civil Rights Act
    c. OSHA
    d. Equal Pay Act
    e. HIPAA

LEARNING APPLICATION

Critical Thinking

1. You have just accepted a position to work in a larger, more specialized clinic where you will be able to use skills you are not currently able to exercise. Identify two or three main points for the letter of resignation you will prepare.

____

____

____

____

2. An employee approaches you, the HR manager, identifying that he or she has just become responsible for the care of an aging parent and may require occasional time away from work. You have no policy about how this absence should be treated. What kind of policy might be helpful? Where would you look for suggestions?

____

____

____

____

____

3. An exit interview form has been introduced in this chapter. Another simple form for an exit interview is to use the ABCs—A stands for "awesome." What do we do that is awesome? B stands for "better." What could we do better in our organization? C stands for "change." What would you recommend we change? Discuss the merits of both forms for an exit interview.

4. What might employers and HR managers do to make certain they keep valued employees? Is salary really the most important issue?

5. As a student preparing for employment, identify what you would need to apply for a position using each of the following avenues for employment: LinkedIn, Facebook, newspaper ads, and Craigslist. For each, identify a minimum of two personal or professional characteristics you will choose to highlight.

Case Studies

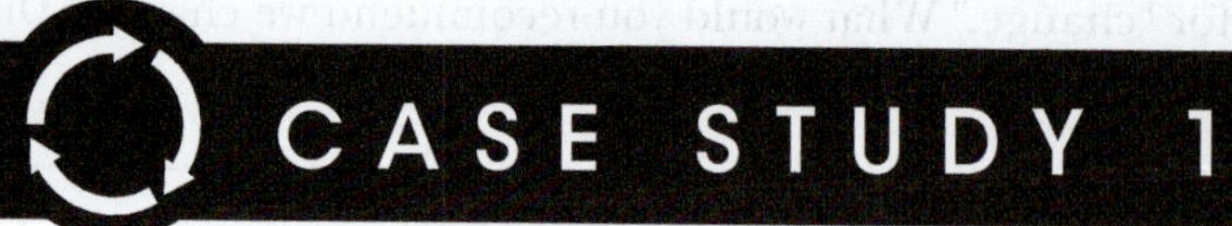

Since Inner City Health Care has expanded to cover a rapidly growing patient load, including the hiring of a co-clinic manager and a new clinical medical assistant, the work pace has been hectic, but challenging. At the suggestion of Dr. Lewis, the clinic managers decide to hold a staff meeting to talk about ways to keep the lines of communication open and to process the many changes occurring at the growing medical practice. Marilyn Johnson, CMA (AAMA), and Jane O'Hara, RMA (AMT), encourage staff to be vocal with their feedback, suggestions, and concerns.

CASE STUDY REVIEW QUESTIONS

1. What other techniques can the clinic managers use to prevent or solve conflicts in the workplace during the period of growth and transition?

____

____

____

____

____

____

____

2. Why is effective communication one of the most important goals of the HR manager?

____

____

ATTRIBUTES OF PROFESSIONALISM

1. This chapter provides good information and insight into the hiring process. If you were put into the position of hiring a new employee, what Attributes of Professionalism would you be looking for? In your journal, make a list of the technical skills your new employee would need and a list of the affective (behavior) skills your new employee would need, including a positive attitude, a good work ethic, and so forth.
   - Determine how you could measure the technical skills you listed.
   - Determine how you could quantify the affective (behavior) skills you listed above.
   - How could you determine those qualities?
   - Which is more difficult to measure: technical or behavioral qualities? Which is more difficult to teach?

____

____

____

2. After completing the preceding scenarios, think about your own interview for a position as medical assistant. When you interview for a job, what technical and behavioral skills on your lists will you need to improve on? Incorporate the Attributes of Professionalism, being realistic and honest.

____

____

____

Name ____________ Date ________ Score ________

CHAPTER 46

Preparing for Medical Assisting Credentials

VOCABULARY BUILDER

Matching

Match each vocabulary term to the aspect of the certification process that best describes it.

________	1. Certification examination	A.	Method for earning points toward recertification
________	2. Certified medical assistant (CMA [AAMA])	B.	A standardized means of evaluating medical assistant competency
________	3. Continued education units (CEUs)	C.	Maintaining current certification status
________	4. Certified clinical medical assistant (CCMA)	D.	Credential awarded for successfully passing the AAMA certification examination
________	5. Recertification	E.	Credential awarded for successfully passing the AMT examination
________	6. Registered medical assistant (RMA)	F.	One of the credentials awarded for passing the National Healthcare Association exam

LEARNING REVIEW

Short Answer

1. Name the three major areas tested in the AAMA certification examination and describe what each includes.

2. List the contact information (addresses, telephone numbers, and Web sites) for obtaining applications for the certification examinations of the AAMA, AMT, and NHA. (Hint: Access each organization's Web site to obtain the most current information.)

AAMA

AMT

NHA

3. To keep their CMA (AAMA) credentials current, how often are individuals required to recertify? How many continuing education units (CEUs) are necessary to recertify?

4. What are the criteria that have been established for applicants to be able to sit for the RMA examination?

5. In addition to the RMA credential, what is the credential that the AMT offers for those who primarily want to be employed in the front offices of provider offices, clinics, or hospitals?

6. List the criteria an applicant must possess to take the NHA certification exam.

____

____

____

____

CERTIFICATION REVIEW

These questions are designed to mimic the certification examination. Select the best response.

1. On the General Medical Assisting Knowledge portion of the AMT certification examination, what besides anatomy and physiology and medical terminology is covered?
   a. Insurance and billing
   b. Medical ethics
   c. Book-keeping and filing
   d. First aid

2. How many multiple-choice questions are on the AMT registration exam?
   a. 300
   b. 250
   c. 210
   d. 310
   e. 500

3. A total of how many questions are on the CMA (AAMA) certification examination?
   a. 100
   b. 200
   c. 1,000
   d. It varies year to year

4. How often does an RMA need to recertify?
   a. Every year
   b. Every 6 years
   c. Every 5 years
   d. Every 3 years
   e. Upon reaching the required 35 points

5. A total of how many CEUs are required to recertify the CMA (AAMA) credential?
   a. 45
   b. 60
   c. 100
   d. 120

6. When recertifying through the AAMA, a minimum of how many units is required in each of the three categories?
   a. 15
   b. 20
   c. 10
   d. 30
   e. 25

7. What is the purpose of certification?
   a. It acknowledges that you are a professional with standard entry-level knowledge and skills.
   b. It builds your personal self-esteem and confidence in knowing that you can do the job asked of you.
   c. It helps in your career advancement and compensation.
   d. All of the above

8. What does the acronym CAAHEP stand for?
   a. Commission Addressing Allied Health Education Programs
   b. Certification and Accreditation of Allied Health Education Programs
   c. Commission on Accreditation of Allied Health Education Programs
   d. Certification for Addressing Allied Health Education Programs
   e. Commission for Addressing Accreditation of Health Education Programs

9. What does the acronym ABHES stand for?
   a. Accrediting Bureau of Health Education Schools
   b. Application Body for Health Education Schools
   c. Application Bureau of Health Education Schools
   d. Accrediting Body of Health Education Schools

10. Which of the following topics is not part of the General Medical Assisting Knowledge portion of the RMA (AMT) exam?
    a. Anatomy and physiology
    b. Patient education
    c. Medical terminology
    d. Asepsis
    e. Human relations

LEARNING APPLICATION

Critical Thinking

1. You are a recent high school graduate and have decided to pursue medical assisting as a career. What will you do to find a school offering an accredited program? Is accreditation important? How might your school selection impact your future as a professional medical assistant?

2. After graduation from your medical assisting program, you plan to sit for a certification examination. How will you prepare for the examination to ensure a positive outcome and earn your CMA/RMA credential?

3. After graduating from an accredited medical assisting program, you immediately went to work as a medical assistant. Now that you have been working several years you decide to become credentialed. How will you achieve this?

Case Studies

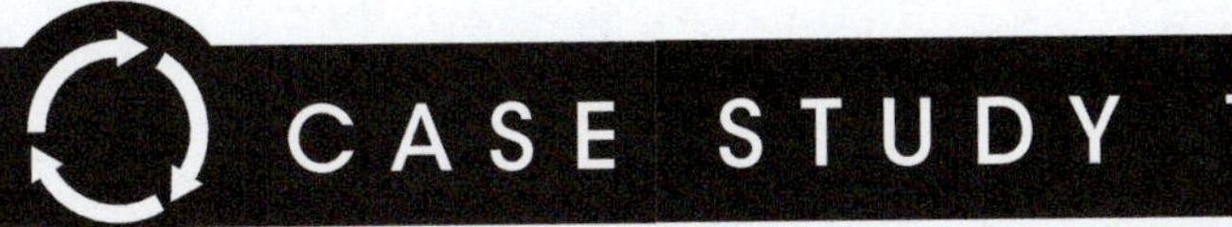

Michele Lucas is performing her practicum at Inner City Health Care under the direction of clinic manager Marilyn Johnson, CMA (AAMA). Michele has purchased a certification review study guide and has taken the sample 120-question certification examination available from the AAMA. From her studies, she has determined that she needs more work in the areas of collections and insurance processing. Administrative medical assistant Ellen Armstrong, CMAS (AMT), is responsible for these duties at Inner City Health Care, under Marilyn's supervision.

CASE STUDY REVIEW QUESTIONS

1. How can Michele use her practicum experience to help her concentrate on improving her skills in the area of collections and insurance processing?

____

____

____

____

____

2. What are your own personal strengths and weaknesses related to preparing for a certification examination through AAMA, AMT, or NHA? What can you do to improve your areas of weakness?

____

____

ATTRIBUTES OF PROFESSIONALISM

Earning a medical assisting credential requires competency and initiative. The following activities will aid you in accomplishing your long-term goal of becoming a credentialed medical assistant.

1. Think of two different places where you could get continuing education credits.
   a. Investigate each one.
   b. Write a paragraph on the benefits and disadvantages of each method for you and your lifestyle.
2. Find out when and where your local chapter meetings of the credentialing organization are held.
   a. Attend a meeting with a classmate.
   b. Discuss what you learned from the meeting.
3. What can you do to prepare for the national certification examination?
   a. Write a plan in which you determine how much time you have to prepare and what you will accomplish each week/month in preparation.
   b. Make a calendar showing the steps toward your examination.
   c. Try to stick with the plan as you progress closer to the examination date.

Name ______________________ Date ________ Score ________

CHAPTER 47

Employment Strategies

VOCABULARY BUILDER

Misspelled Words

Find the words listed below that are misspelled; circle them, and correctly spell them in the spaces provided. Then match each correct vocabulary term to the aspect of the job-seeking process that best describes it.

accomplishment statements
application form
carreer objective
contact tracker
cover letter
cronologic résumé
functional résumé
intervue
refrences
résumé
targeted résumé

______________________ ______________________ ______________________

______________________ ______________________ ______________________

______________________ 1. Expresses your career goal and the position for which you are applying

______________________ 2. Résumé format used to highlight specialty areas of accomplishments and strengths

______________________ 3. A form devised by a prospective employer to collect information relative to qualifications, education, and experience in employment

______________________ 4. Individuals who have known or worked with you long enough to make an honest assessment and recommendation regarding your employment history and qualifications

______________________ 5. Résumé format used when focusing on a clear, specific job

______________________ 6. Statements that begin with a power verb and give a brief description of what you did and the demonstrable results that were produced

______________________ 7. A brief presentation of your qualifications and experience in your chosen career

______________________ 8. A letter used to introduce yourself and your résumé to a prospective employer in response to an unsolicited application or job posting, with the goal of obtaining an interview

______________ 9. Résumé format used when you have employment experience

______________ 10. A meeting in which you discuss employment opportunities within a particular organization and strengths that you can bring to the organization

______________ 11. Form used to keep track of employment contact information, such as name of employer, name of contact person, address and telephone number, date of first contact, résumé sent, interview date, and follow-up information and dates

LEARNING REVIEW

Short Answer

1. List three types of professionals that would make excellent reference choices.

____

2. Identify individuals that you know personally, or have some contact with, who fit each professional reference type you listed above, and explain why you think they would be excellent references for you.

____

____

3. Identify the situations in which using a targeted résumé is advantageous by circling the number next to the statements that apply.
   a. You are just starting your career and have little experience, but you know what you want and you are clear about your capabilities.
   b. You want to use one résumé for several different applications.
   c. You are not clear about your abilities and accomplishments.
   d. You can go in several directions, and you want a different résumé for each.
   e. You are able to keep your résumé on a computer or flash drive.

4. Identify the situations in which using a chronologic résumé is advantageous by circling the number next to the statements that apply.
   a. The position is in a highly traditional field.
   b. Your job history shows real growth and development.
   c. You are changing career goals.
   d. You are looking for your first job.
   e. You are staying in the same field as prior jobs.

5. Identify the situations in which using a functional résumé is advantageous by circling the number next to the statements that apply.
   a. You have extensive specialized experience.
   b. Your most recent employers have been highly prestigious.
   c. You have had a variety of different, apparently unconnected, work experiences.
   d. You want to emphasize a management growth pattern.
   e. Much of your work has been volunteer, freelance, or temporary.

6. List four items that are important when completing a job application.

____

____

____

____

7. Bob Thompson has an interview at Inner City Health Care for a new clinical medical assisting position. He is confident that he has prepared well for the interview. On the way to the interview, Bob reminds himself of three principles he has learned about interviewing:
   a. ______ before answering questions, and try to provide the information requested in a professional manner
   b. ______ carefully so that you understand what information the interviewer is requesting
   c. ________________ if you are uncertain

8. How would you "dress for success" when preparing for your interview?

____

____

____

____

____

CERTIFICATION REVIEW

These questions are designed to mimic the certification examination. Select the best response.

1. Telling your friends, family, personal provider, dentist, and ophthalmologist that you are looking for a position in health care is called what?
   a. Networking
   b. References
   c. Professionalism
   d. Critiquing

2. One important quality an employer looks for in employees is what?
   a. How close they live to the clinic
   b. How many children they have
   c. Their attitude
   d. The number of previous jobs in the health care field
   e. Relationship to other employees

3. What type of résumé should be developed by someone who is just starting a career and has little experience?
   a. Targeted résumé
   b. Chronologic résumé
   c. Functional résumé
   d. Objective résumé

4. Poise includes which of the following attributes?
   a. Skill level
   b. Confidence and professional appearance
   c. Stable mannerisms
   d. The ability to multitask
   e. Both a and b

5. Providing a second opportunity to express your interest in an organization and a position may be done with which of the following?
   a. Cover letter
   b. Recommendation letter
   c. Follow-up letter
   d. Strategic letter

6. A positive and professional attitude is reflected in which of the following reactions in the workplace?
   a. Taking direction
   b. Seeking excellence or doing just enough to get by
   c. Assuming responsibility for your actions and considering your problems not to be someone else's fault
   d. Meeting your employer's needs, not just looking forward to payday
   e. All of the above

7. Some examples of transferable skills include which of the following? *(circle all that apply)*
   a. Leadership
   b. Communication
   c. Keyboarding
   d. Drawing blood

8. What should you do when using someone as a reference?
   a. Always ask permission first, before the name is printed on the reference list
   b. Use your relatives
   c. Verify correct spelling, title, place of employment and position, and telephone number
   d. Ask them to embellish your work experience
   e. Both a and c

9. Which of the following are costly errors that some people make on their résumés?
   a. Typographical and grammatical errors
   b. Mentioning jobs that have transferable skills
   c. Truthfulness
   d. All of the above

10. During the initial interview, what question(s) would be considered *not* appropriate for you to ask?
   a. If this is a newly created position
   b. If there are opportunities for advancement with this organization
   c. About salary, sick leave, benefits, or vacation
   d. What the interviewer considers to be the most difficult task on the job
   e. Whether the last person in this position was promoted

LEARNING APPLICATION

Critical Thinking

1. Discuss the various résumé styles with a classmate and how to determine which style best presents your knowledge and skills to a prospective employer.

2. After reading the section discussing methods of researching a prospective employer, how will you proceed with your research?

Case Studies

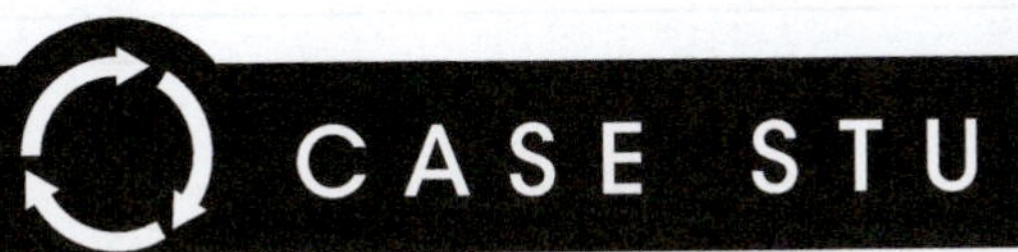

CASE STUDY REVIEW QUESTION

1. You are the subject of this case study. Complete the Self-Evaluation Worksheet that follows. Use your answers to help you determine the working environment you are most interested in and that best suits you. The worksheet can become a useful tool when researching prospective employers to target for your exciting first job in the medical assisting profession.

SELF-EVALUATION WORKSHEET

Respond to the following questions honestly and sincerely. They are meant to assist you in self-assessment.

1. List your three strongest professional attributes:
   a. ___________
   b. ___________
   c. ___________
2. List your three weakest professional attributes:
   a. ___________
   b. ___________
   c. ___________
3. How well do you express yourself? List some examples.
   Orally ___________
   In writing ___________
4. Do you work well as a leader of a group or team? Yes ___________ No ___________
5. Do you prefer to work alone and on your own? Yes ___________ No ___________
6. Can you work under stress/pressure? Yes ___________ No ___________
7. Do you enjoy new ideas and situations? Yes ___________ No ___________
8. Are you comfortable with routines/schedules? Yes ___________ No ___________
9. Which work setting do you prefer?
   Single-provider ___________ Multiprovider ___________
   Small clinic ___________ Large clinic ___________
   Single-specialty ___________ Multispecialty ___________
10. Are you willing to relocate? ___________ Willing to travel? ___________

____

____

Application Activities

1. In the case study, you completed a self-assessment form to help you find the type of working environment that you are most interested in and that best suits you. Create a contact tracker file for yourself, based on the one shown in Figure 47-1 in your textbook. Compile a list from the Internet, want ads in your local paper, your program director, and other sources. (Hint: Other sources are listed in the textbook.)
2. Refer to the "Typical Questions Asked During an Interview" Quick Reference Guide in your textbook (page 1490). Write what you would say to a potential employer in response to all of these questions. Then role-play with another student, acting as interviewer and interviewee, with these questions and answers to gain confidence for an interview.
3. Recall that the interview process is a "two-way street." You, as the interviewee, should interview the employer. The text lists several example questions you might ask the interviewer during an interview. Develop a list of at least two additional questions that are important to you during the interview process.

ATTRIBUTES OF PROFESSIONALISM

As you embark on your new career as a medical assistant, think about how the Attributes of Professionalism will help you in your search for work.

1. List examples of how you would exhibit attributes of professionalism during the interview process and land that dream job.
   a. Examples of communication: ______________________________
   ____
   b. Examples of presentation: ______________________________
   ____
   c. Examples of competency: ______________________________
   ____
   d. Examples of initiative: ______________________________
   ____
   e. Examples of integrity: ______________________________
   ____

____

Comprehensive Examination

1. Which term describes false and malicious writing about another that constitutes defamation of character?
   a. Slander
   b. Assault
   c. Libel
   d. Invasion of privacy
   e. Battery

2. What stage of grief is present when patients cannot believe they are dying?
   a. Denial
   b. Depression
   c. Bargaining
   d. Acceptance
   e. Aggression

3. What document allows an individual to make decisions related to health care when the patient is no longer able to do so?
   a. Living will
   b. Durable power of attorney for health care
   c. Health care directive
   d. DNR order
   e. Specific authorization for health care

4. What document will inform loved ones of the patient's decision related to whether he or she wishes their life to be prolonged in case of medical emergency?
   a. Health care directive
   b. Medical power of attorney
   c. DNR order
   d. Durable power of attorney for health care
   e. Specific health care authorization

5. Which of the following health care professionals are licensed by each state to prepare and dispense all types of medications as well as medical supplies related to medication administration?
   a. Nurse practitioners
   b. Medical illustrators
   c. Pharmacists
   d. Clinical laboratory technicians
   e. Certified medical assistants

6. Which legal principle is violated when a medical assistant practices outside his or her training?
   a. Public duty
   b. Consent
   c. Privacy rights
   d. Confidentiality
   e. Standard of care

7. Which manner of dress is appropriate for an interview?
   a. A medical assistant's uniform
   b. Evening makeup
   c. Spectacular nail polish
   d. Casual clothing
   e. Neat business attire

8. A medical assistant must *never* do which of the following?
   a. Perform a venipuncture
   b. Perform a laboratory test
   c. Imply that he or she is a nurse
   d. Dispense a medication after a direct order from the provider
   e. Give a medication after a direct order from the provider

9. All states require physician assistants to complete an accredited, formal education program and to pass the Physician Assistant National Certifying Examination. Which of the following administers the exam required by all states for licensure of physician assistants?
   a. NCCPA
   b. NCLEX
   c. ABHES
   d. ARNP
   e. CMA-PA

10. Which provider is the most likely to evaluate and treat medical conditions that result from trauma or sudden illness?
    a. Primary care physician
    b. Emergency medical doctor
    c. General practitioner
    d. Family practitioner
    e. Hospitalist

11. What is the purpose of the certification credential for medical assistants?
    a. The certification credential is required for graduation.
    b. The certification credential guarantees a job.
    c. The certification credential meets state registration requirements.
    d. The certification credential indicates a medical assistant's professional and technical competence.
    e. The certification credential meets state licensure requirements.

12. What health care professional develops activity plans for each individual that integrate a complete approach to fitness and wellness through exercise, strength training, and proper diet?
    a. Occupational therapist
    b. Registered dietician
    c. Athletic trainer
    d. Personal fitness trainer
    e. Pilates and yoga instructor

13. What type of people let events, other people, or environmental factors dictate their behavior?
   a. Outer-directed people
   b. Inner-directed people
   c. Micromanagers
   d. Combative people
   e. Assertive people

14. What is the name the psychological term for the experience of long-term emotional, mental, and physical exhaustion?
   a. Goals
   b. Self-actualization
   c. Burnout
   d. Depression
   e. Kinetics

15. What body system reacts to fight-or-flight stress where the large muscles and heart muscles dilate to increase blood flow?
   a. Nervous
   b. Respiratory
   c. Cardiovascular
   d. Endocrine
   e. Musculoskeletal

16. Which statement is accurate regarding the Americans with Disabilities Act (ADA)?
   a. The ADA applies only to medical practices and health care facilities.
   b. The ADA applies to all businesses.
   c. The ADA applies only to businesses with 15 or more employees.
   d. The ADA applies only to businesses with 50 or more employees.
   e. The ADA applies only to state and federal government agencies.

17. What is identified as the "clinical response" to the signs and symptoms of increased or decreased appetite, sleep disorders (insomnia, nightmares), nervous habits (fidgeting, feet tapping, nail biting, pacing, procrastinating or neglecting responsibilities), and lies or excuses to cover up poor work?
   a. Emotional
   b. Physical
   c. Behavioral
   d. Cognitive
   e. All of the above

18. The certifying board of which organization awards the CMA credential?
   a. AAMA
   b. AMT
   c. ABHES
   d. CAAHEP
   e. RMA

19. What involves being aware of what the patient is not saying, or picking up on hints to the real message by observing body language?
    a. Therapeutic communication
    b. Decoding
    c. Active listening
    d. Encoding
    e. Interpreting
20. Which of the following is *not* one of the five Cs of communication?
    a. Clarity
    b. Coherent
    c. Complete
    d. Concise
    e. Courteous
21. What is the highest level in Maslow's Hierarchy of Needs?
    a. Safety needs
    b. Love needs
    c. Self-actualization
    d. Belongingness needs
    e. Esteem needs
22. Which of the following information is considered to be public domain?
    a. A person's sexual preference
    b. A person's police record
    c. A person's past drug addiction
    d. A person's HIV-positive status
    e. A person's alcoholism
23. What is the conscious awareness of one's own feelings and the feelings of others known as?
    a. Congruency
    b. Bias
    c. Self-esteem
    d. Perception
    e. Masking
24. Which best describes the pattern of many concepts, beliefs, values, habits, skills, instruments, and art of a given group of people in a given period?
    a. Culture
    b. Lifestyle
    c. Ideology
    d. Compensation
    e. Comprehension

25. An individual who has done something that results in damage to another person or his or her property would be prosecuted under what type of law?
    a. Statute
    b. Case
    c. Breach of contract
    d. Tort
    e. Regulatory

26. Which of the following would *not* be considered an intentional tort?
    a. Defamation of character
    b. Invasion of privacy
    c. Assault
    d. Negligence
    e. Fraud

27. Oral testimony taken with a court reporter present in a location agreed on by both parties is known as what?
    a. Mediation
    b. Deposition
    c. Interrogatory
    d. Arbitration
    e. *Res ipsa loquitor*

28. What is the legal term that describes a patient who is found by a court to be insane, inadequate, or to not be an adult?
    a. Incompetence
    b. Immaturity
    c. Emancipation
    d. Consent
    e. Immature minor

29. The failure to exercise the standard of care that a reasonable person would exercise in similar circumstances is known as what?
    a. Libel
    b. Slander
    c. Negligence
    d. Malpractice
    e. Extreme carelessness

30. An order for a physician to appear in court with a medical record is known as what?
    a. *Res ipsa loquitur*
    b. *Subpoena duces tecum*
    c. *Respondeat superior*
    d. Interrogatory
    e. Deposition

31. According to the AAMA Code of Ethics, which of the following is a question that medical assistants should ask themselves in order to uphold the honor and high principles of the profession and its disciplines?
    a. Will I give my full attention to acknowledging the needs of every patient?
    b. Will I refrain from needless comments to a colleague regarding a patient's problems?
    c. Will I encourage others to enter the profession and always speak honorably of medical assistants?
    d. Will I honor each patient's request for information and explain unfamiliar procedures?
    e. Will I always perform to the best of my ability, above and beyond the scope of practice of my profession?

32. Which of the following is a term meaning sexual activity between family members?
    a. Intimate partner violence
    b. Incest
    c. Physical abuse
    d. Sexual abuse
    e. Consensual rape

33. What is another term used when describing ethics?
    a. Choices
    b. Beliefs
    c. Morals
    d. Standards
    e. Integrity

34. The majority of states have enacted legislation regarding the abuse of elder adults of what age and older?
    a. 60
    b. 62
    c. 65
    d. 70
    e. 75

35. What is the term used to describe either a place of residence for those who are dying or an organization whose medical professionals and volunteers are in attendance of someone whose death is imminent?
    a. Home health
    b. Rehabilitation
    c. Skilled nursing facility
    d. Hospice
    e. Palliative care

36. The acronym NHA stands for what?
    a. National Health Association
    b. National Healthcareer Association
    c. National Hospital Association
    d. National Hospital Accreditation
    e. Nonprofit Health Alliance

37. The American Medical Technologists (AMT) offers examinations to certify which credential?
    a. CMA
    b. RMA
    c. AAMA
    d. CEU
    e. AMA

38. Only graduates of CAAHEP-accredited and which other medical assisting program(s) may sit for the Certified Medical Assistant exam?
    a. NHA
    b. AAMA
    c. ABHES
    d. CMAS
    e. All of the above

39. Who formulates the AAMA certification examination questions?
    a. TFTC
    b. NHA
    c. CAAHEP
    d. ABHES
    e. AMA

40. What are properties owned by a business, such as supplies and equipment, known as?
    a. Liabilities
    b. Assets
    c. Owner's equity
    d. Accounts
    e. REITs

41. What is the purpose of cost analysis?
    a. To determine the costs of each service
    b. To determine fixed costs
    c. To reduce variable costs
    d. To reduce fixed costs
    e. To determine net profit

42. What should financial records provide to the clinic?
    a. Amount collected in a given period
    b. Amount earned in a given period
    c. Where expenses were incurred in a given period
    d. Financial health of the clinic
    e. All of the above

43. Which of the following is an itemized statement of the assets, liabilities, and owner's equity of a medical facility as of a specified date?
   a. Cost analysis
   b. Accrual basis
   c. Accounting ledger
   d. Income statement
   e. Balance sheet
44. Which of the following is true of the Truth-in-Lending Act?
   a. Providers cannot charge more than 10% interest on their patient accounts.
   b. Providers must charge interest if the account is more than four months past due.
   c. Providers must notify patients in writing if interest is to be charged on their accounts.
   d. If the provider and patient agree to an installment plan of more than four payments, the installment charge must be stated in writing.
   e. Providers must wait at least 3 months before attempting to collect against Medicare patients.
45. When is the best opportunity for collection of amounts due?
   a. One month after the time of service
   b. At the time of service
   c. When cycle billing is performed for the month
   d. After the insurance company has paid its portion of the claim
   e. When the account is sent to a collection agency
46. Management consultants recommend collecting at least a portion of the fees at the time of service and a collection ratio of what percentage?
   a. 50
   b. 80
   c. 85
   d. 90
   e. 95
47. In most states, a debtor may be contacted only between what hours?
   a. 9 AM and 9 PM
   b. 8 AM and 9 PM
   c. 8 AM and 8 PM
   d. 9 AM and 10 PM
   e. 9 AM and 7 PM
48. What is the name of the form that patients with Medicare must sign and is the only legal means a clinic has to collect payment on charges not allowed by Medicare?
   a. Advanced Patient Notice
   b. Advanced Charge Notice
   c. Advanced Beneficiary Notice
   d. Advanced Payment Notice
   e. Advanced Health Care Directive

49. What is an advantage to the ambulatory care setting that accepts credit/debit cards for fees charged?
   a. Minimal amounts of usage
   b. Funds available within 24 hours
   c. Funds available within 48 hours
   d. Instantaneous deposit to clinic account
   e. Service charge on each transaction

50. On a patient account or ledger, where is the credit column located?
   a. On the right and is used for entering charges
   b. On the left and shows the amount due
   c. On the right and is used for entering payments
   d. On the right and shows the amount due
   e. None of the above

51. The amount of cash on hand for the purpose of petty cash is usually within what range?
   a. $75 to $100
   b. $85 to $125
   c. $50 to $150
   d. $50 to $100
   e. $200

52. What does the acronym HCPCS stand for?
   a. Health Common Procedure Code System
   b. Healthcare Common Procedure Coding System
   c. Health Care Classification Procedural Coding System
   d. Healthcare Common Permanent Code Solution
   e. Health Care Provisional Coding Solution

53. What does the acronym CPT stand for?
   a. Comprehensive Patient Treatments
   b. Current Procedural Terminology
   c. Curative Procedures Tried
   d. Curative Patient Treatments
   e. Comprehensive Patient Terminology

54. What does the acronym ICD stand for?
   a. Incidental Codes of Diagnosis
   b. Internal Codes for Decisions
   c. International Codes for Diagnosis
   d. Internal Coding for Diseases
   e. International Classification of Diseases

55. What is an individual who receives Medicare referred to as for insurance purposes?
   a. Beneficiary
   b. Claimant
   c. Policy owner
   d. Individual
   e. Group member

56. What was the original intent of the managed care organization (MCO) model in addition to providing for more efficient use of medical resources?
    a. Control treatment plans
    b. Curb medical costs
    c. Avoid conflicts of interest
    d. Recognize a profit
    e. Keep all health care with one provider

57. Outpatient expenses such as physical therapy, laboratory tests, ambulance services, and charges for durable medical equipment (DME) are covered by which "part" of Medicare?
    a. Part A
    b. Part B
    c. Part C
    d. Part D
    e. Part E

58. Which of the following is true about a coordination of benefits?
    a. A referral is always required.
    b. A deductible does not apply.
    c. The final total benefit is greater than the original charge.
    d. Rules follow a set of guidelines by NAIC to avoid duplicate payment for medical services when there are two policies.
    e. Rules follow a set of guidelines by NDC to avoid duplicate payment for medical services when there are two family members on the same policy.

59. What is the name for the sac that covers the heart?
    a. Pericardium
    b. Epicardium
    c. Endocardium
    d. Myocardium
    e. Mediastinum

60. What structure is responsible for the formation of urine?
    a. Medulla
    b. Cortex
    c. Nephron
    d. Major calyx
    e. Minor calyx

61. What is the name of a congenital disorder that involves one or more vertebrae?
    a. Cerebral palsy
    b. Muscular dystrophy
    c. Tay–Sachs disease
    d. Spina bifida
    e. Hydrocele

62. Which of the following is a characteristic of a malignant tumor?
    a. Smooth borders
    b. Irregular shape
    c. Slow growth
    d. Well-differentiated cells
    e. Encapsulation

63. What is the name for muscular movements that are out of conscious control (e.g., the heart beating)?
    a. Voluntary
    b. Involuntary
    c. Agonist
    d. Antagonist
    e. Synergistic

64. What type of joint allows for the greatest range of motion?
    a. Hinge
    b. Suture
    c. Pivot
    d. Cartilaginous
    e. Ball and socket

65. What portion of the brain is responsible for higher thought processes such as logical thinking?
    a. Parietal lobe
    b. Frontal lobe
    c. Occipital lobe
    d. Temporal lobe
    e. Cerebellum

66. An individual with a blood type of O positive is considered what?
    a. A universal recipient
    b. An ineligible donor
    c. A donor who can donate only to people with O positive blood
    d. A donor who can donate only to people with only O negative blood
    e. A universal donor

67. Which of the following describes the type of immunity that is developed from being vaccinated?
    a. It is naturally acquired active immunity.
    b. It is artificially acquired passive immunity.
    c. It is artificially acquired active immunity.
    d. It is naturally acquired passive immunity.
    e. It is naturally acquired active passive immunity.

68. An X-ray study that is shot from the back of the person toward the front would be considered what?
    a. AP
    b. Lateral
    c. Oblique
    d. PA
    e. Transverse

69. Which of the following is *not* a portion of the large intestine?
    a. Duodenum
    b. Cecum
    c. Transverse colon
    d. Rectum
    e. Ascending colon

70. When performing screenings, the medical assistant must do which of the following?
    a. Diagnose patients' symptoms
    b. Prioritize patients' needs
    c. Allow patients to determine their own needs
    d. Schedule patients in the order in which they arrive
    e. Evaluate patients' ability to pay

71. A person with a hypersensitivity to a bee sting may go into what?
    a. Cardiac arrest
    b. Neurogenic shock
    c. Anaphylactic shock
    d. Seizures
    e. Respiratory shock

72. All of the following statements about shock are accurate *except* what?
    a. There is inadequate circulation to body parts.
    b. The patient's body is kept warm to prevent chilling.
    c. The patient's pulse becomes rapid and weak.
    d. The medical assistant can administer medication as ordered by the provider.
    e. The patient's blood pressure increases.

73. What percentage do most traditional insurance plans have as a co-insurance amount?
    a. 70 to 80
    b. 100
    c. 50 to 60
    d. 60 to 70
    e. 90 to 100

74. A reception area does include which of the following?
    a. Be comfortable and inviting
    b. Be clean and uncluttered
    c. Contain current reading materials for all ages
    d. Have a seating ratio of 2.5 seats for each examination room
    e. All of the above

75. You are a medical assistant in an ambulatory care facility, and an emergency situation arises. What should you do first?
    a. Notify the provider
    b. Give first aid
    c. Assess the patient
    d. Call 911
    e. Contact next of kin

76. What is the name for the act of evaluating the urgency of a medical situation and prioritizing treatment?
   a. Screening
   b. Empathy
   c. Trauma
   d. Diagnosing
   e. Triage

77. Which condition is detected with the Mantoux test?
   a. HIV
   b. Syphilis
   c. PKU
   d. TB
   e. Infectious mononucleosis

78. Which of the following is used as a contrast medium for a radiographic lower GI examination?
   a. Air
   b. Iodine salts
   c. Water
   d. A barium swallow
   e. A barium enema

79. Which type of pathogen causes mumps, measles, and chickenpox?
   a. Bacteria
   b. Viruses
   c. Spirochetes
   d. Parasites
   e. Rickettsiae

80. Which body system does the acronym PERRLA refer to?
   a. Cardiovascular
   b. Gastrointestinal
   c. Nervous
   d. Respiratory
   e. Urogenital

81. Which term means difficulty breathing?
   a. Apnea
   b. Bradypnea
   c. Tachypnea
   d. Eupnea
   e. Dyspnea

82. Which of the following statements is accurate regarding vitamins?
   a. Vitamins A, B, D, and E are fat soluble.
   b. Vitamins are needed in large quantities.
   c. Water-soluble vitamins are stored in fatty tissues.
   d. Vitamins are simple molecules.
   e. Vitamins B and C are water soluble.

83. Which statement is accurate regarding ventricular tachycardia?
   a. Ventricular tachycardia causes severe chest pain.
   b. Ventricular tachycardia is life threatening.
   c. Ventricular tachycardia is often seen in patients using depressants.
   d. Ventricular tachycardia has a cardiac cycle that occurs early.
   e. Ventricular tachycardia occurs in healthy people.

84. What action should you take for patients who are very ill, injured, or upset when they arrive at the clinic?
   a. Ask them to reschedule for the end of the clinic day
   b. Ask them to remain in the reception area
   c. Show them to an examination room away from other patients
   d. Immediately refer them to the emergency department at the hospital
   e. Tell them to calm down immediately or the provider cannot examine them

85. Which type of nutrient contains the most calories per gram?
   a. Carbohydrate
   b. Protein
   c. Mineral
   d. Fat
   e. Vitamin

86. Which term describes why a medication should *not* be administered?
   a. Side effect
   b. Contraindication
   c. Potentiation
   d. Idiosyncratic
   e. Cross-tolerance

87. Robby is coming down with chickenpox but does not have any symptoms yet. He is now at what stage?
   a. Acute stage
   b. Convalescent stage
   c. Declining stage
   d. Incubation stage
   e. Prodromal stage

88. Which of the following statements about medical asepsis hand washing is accurate?
   a. Medical assistants should turn the faucet on with a clean, dry paper towel.
   b. Medical assistants should hold their hands upward.
   c. Medical assistants should scrub up to their elbows.
   d. Medical assistants should touch only the inside of the sink with their hands.
   e. Medical assistants should turn off the faucet with a used paper towel.

89. Which of these positions is used for the treatment and examination of the back and buttocks?
   a. Trendelenburg
   b. Dorsal recumbent
   c. Lithotomy
   d. Supine
   e. Prone

90. Which term describes a woman who has never been pregnant?
   a. Multigravida
   b. Nullipara
   c. Nulligravida
   d. Multipara
   e. Primipara

91. Which infection control guidelines are used by all health care professionals for all patients?
   a. Body substance isolation guidelines
   b. Standard Precautions
   c. OSHA guidelines
   d. Transmission-based precautions
   e. Universal Precautions

92. Which of the following is *not* an acceptable wrapping for autoclaving?
   a. Plastic pouches
   b. Muslin
   c. Paper bags
   d. Aluminum foil
   e. Paper wrapping

93. What is the most common disorder of the urinary system?
   a. Renal calculi
   b. Urinary tract infection
   c. Glomerulonephritis
   d. Cystitis
   e. Pyelonephritis

94. Which of the following diseases is transmitted sexually?
   a. Pelvic inflammatory disease
   b. Cervical cancer
   c. Endometriosis
   d. Prostatitis
   e. Ovarian cancer

95. Which term describes an infection of the middle ear?
   a. Otitis externa
   b. Otalgia
   c. Otitis media
   d. Otorrhagia
   e. Otosclerosis

96. Which condition is commonly known as fainting?
   a. Tinnitus
   b. Singultus
   c. Bruit
   d. Syncope
   e. Vertigo

97. Which of the following is a progressive degenerative disease of the liver?
    a. Hepatitis A
    b. Cholecystitis
    c. Hepatomegaly
    d. Hepatitis B
    e. Cirrhosis

98. Which type of injection is made into the fatty layer just below the skin?
    a. Intramuscular
    b. Subcutaneous
    c. Intradermal
    d. Intravenous
    e. Intermuscular

99. An elevation of which blood cell count indicates the presence of inflammation in the body?
    a. Platelet count
    b. Erythrocyte sedimentation rate
    c. Hematocrit
    d. Total hemoglobin
    e. White blood cell differentiation

100. What condition is characterized by an abnormal thickening and hardening of the skin?
    a. Acne
    b. Melanoma
    c. Dermatophytosis
    d. Scleroderma
    e. Psoriasis

101. Who has the responsibility of keeping the reception area clean and organized?
    a. Administrative medical assistant
    b. Bookkeeper
    c. Laboratory technician
    d. Office manager
    e. All of the above

102. Homeostasis refers to what?
    a. Sterile environment
    b. Complete procedure
    c. Everyone getting along
    d. Internal equilibrium
    e. Rapid heart rate

103. What is the classification of drugs with the lowest potential of abuse?
    a. Schedule II
    b. Schedule II
    c. Schedule III
    d. Schedule IV
    e. Schedule V

104. The provider you are working with asks you to provide a patient with samples of a new medication. When you comply, you are doing what?

a. Prescribing medication
b. Administering medication
c. Compounding medication
d. Mixing medication
e. Dispensing medication

105. Which of the following is information about a medication that is *not* found in the PDR?

a. Indications for use
b. Shape of each pill
c. Dosage and administration route
d. Precautions
e. Generic name

106. A drug that increases the effect of another has which type of effect?

a. Local
b. Remote
c. Synergistic
d. Systemic
e. Topical

107. How would a medication that is ordered to be delivered in a sublingual route be administered?

a. Placed in the cheek
b. Swallowed
c. Inserted into the rectum
d. Placed under the tongue
e. Placed on top of the tongue

108. A medication that is classified as an expectorant would have what effect?

a. Dilate bronchi
b. Prevent coughing
c. Relax blood vessels
d. Decrease nausea
e. Increase the amount of mucus being expelled

109. A medication that increases the amount of urine excreted by the body would be classified as what?

a. Diuretic
b. Antiarrhythmic
c. Antiemetic
d. Vasopressor
e. Muscle relaxant

110. All of the following are part of a medication order *except* what?

a. Name of drug
b. Who dispenses the medication
c. Form of drug
d. Route of administration
e. Prescribing provider's signature

111. A prescription that indicates a medication should be administered "OD" would go where?
   a. Left eye
   b. Right ear
   c. Left ear
   d. Right eye
   e. In the nose

112. What is the metric prefix which refers to one-millionth of a unit?
   a. Milli
   b. Kilo
   c. Meter
   d. Gram
   e. Micro

113. Pediatric medication dosages are figured based on what information about the child?
   a. Height
   b. Age
   c. Weight
   d. Gender
   e. Chest circumference

114. A patient weighs 130 pounds. The provider asked you to convert that weight into kilograms. You know that there are 2.2 pounds in 1 kilogram. How many kilograms does this patient weigh?
   a. 4.55 kg
   b. 59.09 kg
   c. 286 kg
   d. 0.07 kg
   e. 260 kg

115. Which of the following is *not* one of the six rights of medication administration?
   a. Dose
   b. Provider
   c. Route
   d. Patient
   e. Drug

116. Parenteral medication is administered via what method?
   a. Mouth
   b. Rectum
   c. Skin
   d. Inhalation
   e. Injection

117. What type of injection is administered at a 90-degree angle?
   a. Subcutaneous
   b. Intradermal
   c. Intravenous
   d. Inhaled
   e. Intramuscular

118. Hypodermic needles are most appropriate for what?
    a. Venipuncture
    b. Aspirations
    c. Allergy injections
    d. Intramuscular and subcutaneous injections
    e. Insulin administration

119. Which of the following is *not* an appropriate injection site for an intramuscular injection?
    a. Dorsogluteal
    b. Biceps
    c. Ventrogluteal
    d. Deltoid
    e. Vastus lateralis

120. Which of the following will a poorly illuminated reception room suggest to patients?
    a. Soiled carpets
    b. Dusty baseboards
    c. Faded draperies
    d. Poor housekeeping
    e. All of the above

121. The keyboard and the mouse are considered to be what kind of devices?
    a. The most common types of input devices
    b. The most common types of output devices
    c. Portable memory storage devices
    d. Read-write devices
    e. The central processing unit

122. What should you do to ensure that your work in the computer is safe from hackers?
    a. Store all work on data storage devices
    b. Defragment frequently
    c. Use firewalls
    d. Back up frequently
    e. Use cloud-based storage

123. What is the "brain" of the computer called?
    a. Motherboard
    b. Modem
    c. Video card
    d. Central processing unit (CPU)
    e. Operating system

124. Which of the following is the most common way to prevent unauthorized use of your clinic computers?
    a. Keep the computer in a locked cabinet at all times
    b. Keep the computer in a locked cabinet at night
    c. Assign every employee a password
    d. Have only one person on the computer at a time
    e. Have screen-savers set to time out at 5 minutes

125. What is the proper term that describes saying words correctly?
 a. Enunciation
 b. Pronunciation
 c. Articulation
 d. Personification
 e. Inflection

126. Which of the following guidelines ensures successful transfer of calls?
 a. Getting the caller's full name, telephone number, and date of birth
 b. Following up to be sure the call transferred directly to the clinic manager
 c. Determining who would be the best person to assist with the situation
 d. Following your telephone system's procedure for transferring the call
 e. Both c and d

127. To whom should a telephone call concerning a complaint about medical service be routed?
 a. Provider
 b. Clinical medical assistant
 c. Administrative medical assistant
 d. File clerk
 e. Risk management department

128. What disease of the eye is characterized by elevated intraocular pressure?
 a. Cataract
 b. Glaucoma
 c. Macular degeneration
 d. Amblyopia
 e. Strabismus

129. What mineral is important for the formation of bone tissue?
 a. Calcium
 b. Potassium
 c. Zinc
 d. Iron
 e. Magnesium

130. Which of the following is a type of bacteria?
 a. Streptococci
 b. Helminth
 c. Protozoa
 d. Tinea
 e. Scabies

131. Diseases caused by which type of pathogen are treated by antibiotics?
 a. Protozoa
 b. Fungi
 c. Bacteria
 d. Virus
 e. Parasite

132. In which situation is personal protective equipment generally *not* necessary?
   a. Handling or processing a urine specimen
   b. Taking vital signs
   c. Performing venipuncture
   d. Assisting with surgical procedures
   e. Disinfecting instruments

133. When prioritizing telephone calls, what is the act of evaluating the urgency of a medical situation?
   a. Screening
   b. Triage
   c. Delegation
   d. Referral
   e. Enunciation

134. Which of the following is an accurate listing of types of scheduling systems?
   a. Wave, modified wave, double booking, mile-a-minute
   b. Open hours, wave, clustering, stream, double booking
   c. First-come, first-served; open hours; clustering
   d. Open hours, closed hours, clustering, double-booking
   e. Wave, first-come/first-served, streaming

135. Use of alcohol-based hand rub is acceptable in which of the following situations?
   a. Before and after eating
   b. Before and after using the restroom
   c. After contact with body excretions
   d. After decontamination of a work area
   e. Following processing of microbiologic specimens

136. Below are guidelines to scheduling. Which one is correct?
   a. Urgent calls should be sent to the hospital, which is better equipped to handle them.
   b. Urgent calls should be assessed before determining the best course of action.
   c. Referrals by other providers need to be seen immediately.
   d. Appointments for pharmaceutical and medical supply representatives should be referred to the provider.
   e. All of the above.

137. Information that should be obtained from all new patients includes all but which of the following?
   a. The patient's full legal name
   b. The patient's birth date
   c. The patient's address and telephone numbers
   d. The patient's insurance information
   e. The patient's family health history

138. When performing CPR on an infant or a child, circulation is checked by assessing pulse at which pulse point?
   a. Carotid
   b. Axial
   c. Femoral
   d. Brachial
   e. Dorsal pedis

139. What method is used to clear an airway obstruction in an unconscious adult?
   a. Finger sweep
   b. Back blows
   c. Chest thrust
   d. Two rescue breaths
   e. CPR

140. A burn that has penetrated to the bone would be considered what?
   a. Superficial
   b. Partial thickness
   c. 100%
   d. Full thickness
   e. 75%

141. Which of the following is *not* a step in controlling bleeding from an open wound on the arm?
   a. Applying direct pressure
   b. Elevating the arm
   c. Wrapping the wound tightly
   d. Applying pressure to the appropriate artery
   e. Disinfecting the area

142. Appropriate first aid for a patient with a case of acute frostbite would include what?
   a. Immersing the area in warm water
   b. Warming the area by creating friction
   c. Immediately raising the patient's core body temperature
   d. Applying heavy moisturizing cream to the area
   e. Immediately debriding necrotic tissues

143. Appropriate treatment for an acute sprain or strain would include all *but* which of the following?
   a. Ice
   b. Rest
   c. Compression
   d. Range of motion
   e. Elevation

144. How would a medication that is to be taken twice a day be indicated?
   a. qd
   b. tid
   c. qid
   d. bid
   e. od

145. Which of the following provides a current and accurate record of appointment times available?
   a. Historical schedule
   b. Patient screening
   c. Appointment matrix
   d. Self-referral
   e. Wave reporting

146. In the SOAPER approach, what does the letter *E* stand for?
    a. Equipment needed
    b. Education for patient
    c. Eliminated medications
    d. Education for staff
    e. Extra reporting

147. Which of the following is *not* an advantage of a manual medical record?
    a. Can be used by only one person at a time
    b. Easier to protect confidentiality
    c. No worry of computer malfunction
    d. Currently established and understood
    e. All of the above

148. Which of the following patients would be filed first if the method of alphabetic filing by last name were used?
    a. Betty Donaldson
    b. Bradley Donalds
    c. Annette Dunn
    d. Abigal Devora
    e. Amber Davidson

149. When names are identical, the patient's address may be used to order files. How is the address indexed?
    a. First – City; Second – State; Third – House number; Fourth - Street name
    b. First – State; Second – City; Third – House number; Fourth - Street name
    c. First – City; Second – State; Third – Street name; Fourth – House number
    d. First – State; Second – House number; Third – City; Fourth – Street name
    e. None of the above – the patient Social Security number is used as the index for order

150. Which of the following is *not* one of the four major letter styles?
    a. Full block
    b. Modified block, standard
    c. Facilitated block
    d. Simplified block
    e. Simplified

151. What part of a letter includes a specially designed logo with the address and phone numbers?
    a. Salutation
    b. Inside address
    c. Letterhead
    d. Reference heading
    e. Enclosure

152. Which of the following is the process of reading a document and checking for accuracy?
    a. Referencing
    b. Proofreading
    c. Verification
    d. Rationalizing
    e. Reference initials

153. Which computerized feature allows you to use a database to send the same letter, although personalized, to many different people?
   a. Word processing letters
   b. Mail merge
   c. Database letters
   d. Merge correspondence
   e. Cloud computing

154. The practice of contracting with a service outside the clinic or hospital to a company where the task can be accomplished at a lower cost and with a faster turnaround time is known as what?
   a. Delegating
   b. Outsourcing
   c. Biometrics
   d. Risk management
   e. Privileged communications

155. What does the abbreviation EMR stands for?
   a. Electronic medical report
   b. Electronic medicine record
   c. Electronic medical record
   d. Electronic medication record
   e. Electric medical record

156. Treating the patient's medical information as private and not for publication is known as which of the following?
   a. Confidentiality
   b. Privacy
   c. Privileged
   d. Concealment
   e. Protocol

157. What is the concise description of the patient's encounter with the medical clinic known as?
   a. Chief complaint
   b. History of present illness
   c. Review of systems
   d. Progress notes
   e. SOAP

158. What does the acronym SDS stand for?
   a. Safety Data Sheet
   b. Safety Documents/Sheets
   c. Standards for Documentation and Safety
   d. Supplies and Data for Safety
   e. Safety Data Summary

159. Which of the following statements is true regarding SDS information?
    a. To be read by all employees
    b. Indexed and alphabetized in a notebook or manual
    c. To be made readily available to all employees
    d. Contains information about chemicals in the workplace
    e. All of the above

160. Which federal agency enforces regulations requiring the labeling of hazardous materials?
    a. CDC
    b. EPA
    c. NFPA
    d. OSHA
    e. CMS

161. Which of the following laboratory tests are *not* PPMP levels of testing?
    a. Urine sediment examinations
    b. Qualitative semen analysis
    c. Urine pregnancy test
    d. Wet mount preparations
    e. Pinworm examinations

162. What microscope is specifically designed for viewing specimens that are transparent and unstained?
    a. Phase-contrast
    b. Fluorescent
    c. Electron
    d. Cytology department
    e. Transparent lucent

163. Which of the following is a description of a panel?
    a. Many tests all billed together at one time
    b. All the tests for one patient during one calendar year
    c. All the tests a doctor orders consistently throughout her or his practice
    d. The blood serum (the part of blood that does not contain cells) tests
    e. The quality controls in place for the lab

164. A low-powered objective lens on a microscope allows the specimen to be magnified to what size for viewing?
    a. 10 times larger than life
    b. 100 times larger than life
    c. 1,000 times larger than life
    d. 10,000 times larger than life
    e. 100,000 times larger than life

165. What is the meaning of the medical abbreviation NPO?
    a. Neuro Plastic Observation
    b. Patient is not to ingest any food
    c. Patient is not to ingest food or drink fluids
    d. Patient is not to drink fluids
    e. None of the above

166. Which of the following produces red blood cells (RBCs)?
   a. Liver
   b. Lymph nodes
   c. Spleen
   d. Kidneys
   e. Bone marrow

167. Which way should the bevel of the needle be held when performing venipuncture?
   a. Up
   b. Down
   c. Sideways
   d. Vertical
   e. Any of the above

168. What is the maximum amount of time a tourniquet should be left on?
   a. 30 seconds
   b. 60 seconds
   c. 90 seconds
   d. 2 minutes
   e. 3 minutes

169. What is the needle gauge size used in blood banking/donations?
   a. 14
   b. 16
   c. 18
   d. 20
   e. 22

170. Which blood cell has the ability to travel through the vessel walls into the tissues?
   a. White blood cells
   b. Red blood cells
   c. Iron-deficient cells
   d. Iron-rich cells
   e. None of the above

171. What is the normal value for the Westergren method of ESR for a female patient older than 50 years?
   a. 0 to 10 mm/hr
   b. 0 to 15 mm/hr
   c. 0 to 20 mm/hr
   d. 0 to 25 mm/hr
   e. 0 to 30 mm/hr

172. Normal blood will clot within what amount of time?
   a. 11 to 13 seconds
   b. 20 to 30 seconds
   c. 45 seconds
   d. 60 seconds
   e. 90 seconds

173. What is the normal number of platelets found in a microliter of blood?
   a. 150 to 4000
   b. 1,500 to 40,000
   c. 150,000 to 400,000
   d. 1,500,000 to 4,000,000
   e. 5,000,000 or more

174. Which part of the urinalysis is to be performed by the provider?
   a. The chemical examination
   b. The physical examination
   c. The specific gravity
   d. The microscopic examination
   e. All of the above

175. What do ketones in urine indicate?
   a. Diabetes
   b. Glomerulonephritis
   c. Lipolysis
   d. A high intake of carbohydrates/sugars
   e. Both a and c

176. What is the most common urine specimen type performed in the provider's office laboratory (POL)?
   a. Sterile specimen
   b. Timed specimen
   c. Random specimen
   d. Catheterized specimen
   e. All of the above

177. Which of the following is *not* a recording of urine transparency?
   a. Clear
   b. Cloudy
   c. Hazy
   d. Musty
   e. Turbid

178. Which of the following is *not* included in the field of microbiology study?
   a. Plants
   b. Bacteria
   c. Fungi
   d. Parasites
   e. Viruses

179. In the microbiology laboratory the term *media* refers which of the following?
   a. The microscopic slide that is smeared with a specimen
   b. The laboratory chemical that is used in testing
   c. A host of substances used to foster the growth of bacteria
   d. A sample of body secretions that contains harmful pathogens
   e. All of the above

180. Appropriate handling of specimens includes which of the following?
 a. Wearing personal protective equipment (PPE)
 b. Washing hands often
 c. Wearing gloves
 d. Never eating, smoking, drinking, or putting objects into the mouth while working with specimens
 e. All of the above

181. What fluid is *not* collected in a sterile specimen container?
 a. Sputum
 b. Urine
 c. Cerebral spinal fluid
 d. Stool specimen
 e. None of the above

182. Source-oriented medical records are organized by what?
 a. The cause of a patient's medical diagnosis
 b. The location of a patient's medical record
 c. The nature of a patient's complaint
 d. The treatment methods being used
 e. The professionals who have documented in the record

183. Which of the following is *not* an example of objective information?
 a. Laboratory data
 b. Diagnosis
 c. Prescribed treatment
 d. Patient's complaint
 e. Examination findings

184. How many different blood types are there?
 a. 3
 b. 5
 c. 4
 d. 6
 e. 8

185. At what time during pregnancy does the hCG level peak?
 a. 5 days after conception
 b. 11 days after conception
 c. 3 to 4 weeks into the pregnancy
 d. 8 to 11 weeks into the pregnancy
 e. Just before delivery

186. What percentage of North Americans are Rh positive?
 a. 20
 b. 35
 c. 50
 d. 65
 e. 85

187. Of the following fats, which one is *not* polyunsaturated?
    a. Olive oil
    b. Corn oil
    c. Sunflower oil
    d. Safflower oil
    e. Fish oil

188. What is known as the slowing of physical and mental responses, decreased alertness, apathy, withdrawal, and diminished interest in work?
    a. Depression
    b. Psychomotor retardation
    c. Mental retardation
    d. Terminal illness
    e. Psychological repression

189. Which of the following is *not* an advantage of a functional résumé?
    a. You want to emphasize a management growth pattern
    b. You are changing careers
    c. You have extensive specialized experience
    d. You are reentering the job market after an absence
    e. Your career path or growth is not clear from a chronologic listing

190. Which type of résumé is best for focusing on a clear, specific job?
    a. Functional
    b. Chronological
    c. Targeted
    d. Basic
    e. Specific

191. What should be listed on a separate sheet of paper that matches your résumé?
    a. Qualifications
    b. Credentials
    c. References
    d. College degrees
    e. Length of employment

192. Exaggerations and lies on your résumé can have serious consequences. Which of the following is considered one of the "Top Ten Serious Lies" on résumés?
    a. Foreign language fluency
    b. Degree received
    c. Professional memberships
    d. Work history
    e. All of the above

193. Which of the following is a characteristic of a leader?
   a. Organizes and allocates talent and resources
   b. Provides vision and goals, setting reasonable and clear standards
   c. Plans and budgets using available resources
   d. Controls and solves problems, with the ability to adapt to changes seamlessly
   e. Consistently achieves goals and targets

194. An office code of conduct is the most helpful preventative measure for which of the following?
   a. Brainstorming
   b. Benchmarking
   c. Conflict resolution
   d. Self-actualization
   e. Performance goals

195. Harassment in the workplace can be in the form of which of the following type of verbal or physical behavior/conduct?
   a. Unwelcome
   b. Based on a protected class
   c. Severe or pervasive
   d. Has a negative impact or creates a hostile environment
   e. All of the above

196. Which of the following is a key point to keep in mind when dismissal of an employee is necessary?
   a. Take no longer than 20 minutes for the dismissal
   b. Escort the employee out of the facility once he or she has finished work for the day
   c. Do not engage in an in-depth conversation of performance
   d. Agree and empathize with all of the employee's opinions and rationalizations
   e. Have at least two witnesses to the dismissal

197. Which of the following must a job description include?
   a. Necessary work experience
   b. Any special certification or licensure
   c. Basic qualifications for the position
   d. Skills and education required
   e. All of the above

198. A suggested item for the interview worksheet would include which of the following?
   a. Ability to problem solve when given a scenario
   b. Description of a work-related decision
   c. Identification of what is most important in a job
   d. Identification of strengths and weaknesses
   e. All of the above

199. What type of action usually occurs when an employee's performance is poor or there has been a serious violation of clinic policies or the job description?
   a. Involuntary dismissal
   b. Voluntary dismissal
   c. Probation
   d. Written advisement
   e. Progressive discipline

200. Which of the following is *not* a question to ask when checking references?
   a. Would you rehire?
   b. Could you describe the position held?
   c. Can you comment on attendance and dependability?
   d. What were the wages of the employee?
   e. What would you consider limitations of the employee?